Register Now f...
to You...

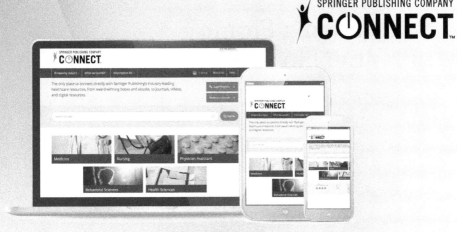

Your print purchase of *Transitioning From LPN/LVN to BSN*, **includes online access to the contents of your book**—increasing accessibility, portability, and searchability!

Access today at:

http://connect.springerpub.com/content/book/978-0-8261-2182-0 or scan the QR code at the right with your smartphone and enter the access code below.

3DU8KXY8

Scan here for quick access.

If you are experiencing problems accessing the digital component of this product, please contact our customer service department at cs@springerpub.com

The online access with your print purchase is available at the publisher's discretion and may be removed at any time without notice.

Publisher's Note: New and used products purchased from third-party sellers are not guaranteed for quality, authenticity, or access to any included digital components.

LS

SPRINGER PUBLISHING COMPANY

View all our products at springerpub.com

Transitioning From LPN/LVN to BSN

Nancy Duphily, DNP, RN-BC, is an accomplished nursing educator and clinical practitioner, having taught and worked in various clinical and educational settings for more than 25 years. She received her BS, MS, and CNS nursing degrees from the University of Massachusetts at Amherst, and her DNP from Regis College, Weston, Massachusetts. She currently serves as assistant professor of nursing at Fitchburg State University, Fitchburg, Massachusetts. She has spent much of her career working as an instructor in LPN programs, and assisting her students in transitioning to more advanced roles. She participated in the introduction of the LPN to BS in nursing program at Fitchburg State University, one of the first in Massachusetts. She is the author of numerous journal articles and professional presentations on various topics in nursing education.

Transitioning From LPN/LVN to BSN

Nancy Duphily, DNP, RN-BC

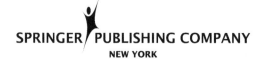
SPRINGER PUBLISHING COMPANY
NEW YORK

Springer Publishing Company, LLC
11 West 42nd Street
New York, NY 10036
www.springerpub.com

Acquisitions Editor: Elizabeth Nieginski
Composition: S4Carlisle Publishing Services
Cover illustration: Bryce Muir (Additional artwork can be viewed at Bryce Muir's website, brycemuir.com, and at the website of the arts center started in his honor, merrymeetingartscenter.org.)
Cover art provided by Jane Page-Conway, Fine Arts Photographer

ISBN: 978-0-8261-2181-3
e-book ISBN: 978-0-8261-2182-0

Qualified instructors may request the Instructor's Manual and PowerPoints by emailing
textbook@springerpub.com
Instructor's Manual ISBN: 978-0-8261-2734-1
PowerPoints ISBN: 978-0-8261-2733-4

14 15 16 17/ 5 4 3 2 1

The author and the publisher of this Work have made every effort to use sources believed to be reliable to provide information that is accurate and compatible with the standards generally accepted at the time of publication. The author and publisher shall not be liable for any special, consequential, or exemplary damages resulting, in whole or in part, from the readers' use of, or reliance on, the information contained in this book. The publisher has no responsibility for the persistence or accuracy of URLs for external or third-party Internet websites referred to in this publication and does not guarantee that any content on such websites is, or will remain, accurate or appropriate.

Library of Congress Cataloging-in-Publication Data

Duphily, Nancy, author.
Transitioning From LPN/LVN to BSN / Nancy Duphily.
    p. ; cm.
Includes bibliographical references and index.
ISBN-13: 978-0-8261-2181-3
ISBN-10: 0-8261-2181-0
ISBN-13: 978-0-8261-2182-0 (e-book)
I. Title.
[DNLM: 1. Nursing. 2. Education, Nursing. 3. Nurse's Role. 4. Nursing Process. WY 101]
RT48
610.73--dc23

2013048891

Printed in the United States of America by Gasch Printing.

Contents

PART IV: SKILL COMPETENCIES FOR THE BACCALAUREATE-PREPARED NURSE

Foreword

This is an exciting time for growth and transformation in the profession of nursing. It is also a call for action in how we infuse new knowledge, develop professionalism, and bridge our knowledge to the practice that is uniquely nursing. Dr. Duphily knows the essential gift that new knowledge brings in the authoring of this book *Transitioning From LPN/LVN to BSN*.

With the publication of the groundbreaking report from the Institute of Medicine released in 2011, *The Future of Nursing: Leading Change, Advancing Health*, we are aware that the health concerns that face our nation and world depend on our profession as nurses working to the highest level of our education. As individuals and as a profession, nurses are called to learn, infuse reflexivity into our practice, apply evidence, and be critical thinkers across complex domains of care. *Transitioning From LPN/LVN to BSN* addresses this call.

This book is a response that fosters education, practice development, and professionalism. The BSN is the essential educational foundation to give nurses the knowledge to improve health outcomes and provide the highest quality care. Contemporary health care delivery requires the nurse's ability to provide care that is culturally competent, patient- and population-centered, technologically advanced, and highly collaborative. Meeting this challenge requires our commitment to professional practice and ongoing education.

Transitioning From LPN/LVN to BSN provides the essentials of nursing theory and the importance of having a philosophy of nursing that informs our professional role. This groundbreaking book for LPN and

LVN education and professional practice transition stresses the important characteristics of the professional nurse as leader, advocate, teacher, manager, and expert communicator. Each chapter offers tools and examples to engage both teachers and students. Dr. Duphily has written this book in her voice, which is supportive and encouraging, and reflects her true passion for teaching, while recognizing the need for the "courage to learn," as Parker Palmer is credited with saying, that is to be fostered in students and one another. In writing this book, Dr. Duphily is leading a professional practice change, and is doing it as a true nurse expert and attentive educator. As an expert nurse, Dr. Duphily encourages us to learn together and often. We are the future of nursing, and sharing this book will effectively guide those seeking to transition into a new professional role that is much needed now and in the future.

Raeann G. LeBlanc, DNP, ANP/GNP-BC
Assistant Clinical Professor
University of Massachusetts Amherst

Preface

When an apple is cut, others see seeds in the apple. We, as nurses, see apples in the seeds.

Martha Rogers, nurse theorist

To both student and educator,

This text is written to assist with the transition from the role of the LPN to the baccalaureate-prepared registered nurse (RN). Emphasis will be placed on the following areas: exploring the role of the RN within the interdisciplinary health care team; describing the experience of returning to the academic setting; and discussion regarding challenges and strategies surrounding areas of successful role acquisition.

Dall'Alba (2009) writes that "learning to become a professional involves not only what we know and can do, but also who we are becoming" (p. 34). Licensed practical nurses (LPNs) who enter a university to advance their education through seeking a baccalaureate of nursing degree often find the experience of socializing into the new professional role challenging. Professional socialization involves acquiring a professional role and evolving as a member of an occupational culture. A significant component of this process is legitimation, the experience of gaining a sense of affirmation from socializing agents (Haas & Shaffir, 1991; Klossner, 2008).

Legitimation is a critical element within the process of professional socialization (Klossner, 2008). It occurs when those around learners affirm that they are actually developing an identity as a member of their chosen profession. As students are professionalized, they are initiated into a new culture wherein they gradually adopt those symbols that represent the profession and its generally accepted authority.

Melrose, Miller, Gordon, and Janzen (2012) examined professional socialization and those socializing agents of legitimation that either enabled or barred the role transition from LPN to baccalaureate-prepared RN. In a descriptive study that explored this experience with professional socialization, the authors explored the socializing factors that contributed to students' feelings of legitimacy in the growth of their new professional identities. Participants were 27 post-LPN to bachelor of science in nursing (BSN) students from a Canadian university who attended a practicum on an acute hospital unit. Focus group methodology enabled the researchers to draw out participants' views and to explore their ideas and conversational exchanges with one another in depth.

Emerging themes illustrated the experience of legitimation among this group of learners. In one of the four themes identified through this study ("Post-LPN to BSN Students Need Little, if Any, Further Legitimation to Affirm Their Identities as 'Nurse'"), participants felt that their identity as a "nurse" was well established before they entered the post-LPN to BSN program: "When I gave my first injection . . . that was like . . . I'm a nurse"; "When clients appreciate the care that you provide them, and also the family, they will speak with you and then thank you for whatever you did"; "I was on the floor as the only official nurse for more than half of my shift . . . with the full responsibility of all 60 residents in my care . . . that all happened as an LPN."

Participants felt their initial LPN education had socialized them into the identity of "nurse." Many felt insulted by the notion of "becoming" a nurse. Given the similarities between the LPN and RN role in their workplaces, they did not always feel that they were doing anything "different" in their practicum. From the post-LPN to BSN students' perspectives, the notion that socialization into the role of "nurse" would occur for them at this point in their career was insulting, as indicated by the following feedback from some students:

> "I almost feel a little bit insulted to think that I would feel any less professional as an LPN than I do as an RN. I feel equally professional in both roles.". . . "We are not newbies, we have been around, and we do bring experience.". . . "I'm still very proud of the work I do as an LPN. I already feel I do think like an RN. [It's] very frustrating and almost devalues the work that I've already put into the profession."

Post-LPN to BSN students in the study expressed that they already viewed themselves as professional nurses. They were not "becoming nurses" by attending a university. One nurse offered this advice to those involved with educating this group of learners: "It's extremely important when you are an adult learner to be treated as such. When you disregard our previous skill and knowledge, it's a blow to our ego, it's degrading."

In another theme ("Practicum Interactions With Instructors and New Clinical Experiences Are Key Socializing Agents"), participants reflected on changes and growth in their professional identity. They credited the practicum interactions with instructors and the opportunities for new experiences as particularly significant. During the practical components of their program, it was especially important to receive legitimation from others that they were truly extending their existing "nurse" identity:

> . . . you need to justify everything that you're doing and explain the reason for it. It makes you think more about your reasons for doing something and whether you can justify them well enough to, you know, proceed to doing care . . . you have somebody who's constantly challenging you to prepare. So if you can give a good answer, you know okay, I'm on the way. What can I do better? If you cannot answer the questions, then you're challenged to go and maybe research a little bit better.

Consistent professional socialization begins when instructors and clients accept students in their new professional role (Klossner, 2008). This acknowledgment by others generates confidence in students, along with a willingness to demonstrate behaviors expected of those in the new role. Research by Spoelstra and Robbins (2010) with RNs transitioning to an advanced practice role reinforces implementing direct patient care as essential to successful role transition.

Implications for both nursing educators and post-LPN to BSN students include respect for the legitimacy (Klossner, 2008) students have already developed as practicing professional nurses. Educators must communicate with students, provide diverse opportunities for learning, and engage learners in topics and experiences that challenge them. Likewise, students are encouraged to seek out their faculty on an ongoing basis in order to keep the lines of communication open, to recognize and address potential problems early on, and to identify individual educational goals for optimal learning.

Traditional undergraduate placements cannot be expected to accommodate all the needs of this diverse group of adult learners. It is critical for educators to recognize that "new" experiences may be different for each student. Knowing the value that this group of adult learners places on instructor evaluation and "new" clinical experiences, implications for educators include ensuring that discussion time between student and teacher is built into the curriculum. Additionally, emphasis should be placed on designing practicum experiences that build on students' established identities as professional nurses (Benner, Sutphen, Leonard, & Day, 2009). At the same time, students' reflections from weekly clinical experiences and placements are extremely valuable in articulating and evaluating which experiences best contribute to and advance their learning.

From the above findings, considering the scarcity of published literature on this topic, and from discussions with practicing LPNs, LPNs in bridge programs, staff nurses, nursing educators, and nursing administrators, this book was written. Their contributions regarding what to include/omit in an LPN to BSN transition program provided its focus; that of supporting this population of nurses who articulate what areas they consider challenging and oftentimes overwhelming in this educational venture.

INTEGRATION OF QUALITY AND SAFETY EDUCATION FOR NURSES (QSEN) STANDARDS

In 2003, the Institute of Medicine issued a challenge to nursing educators to effect fundamental changes in programs to enable graduates to work effectively in a reorganized health care system committed to quality and safety. The Quality and Safety Education for Nurses (QSEN) initiative was formed in 2005 in response to this challenge. From this collaboration, six QSEN standards were created: patient-centered care, teamwork and collaboration, evidence-based practice, quality improvement, safety, and informatics.

At a survey administered during the 2006 National League for Nursing Educational Summit, feedback from attendees revealed that these standards were not being taught. Moreover, faculty did not understand the concepts adequately, and acknowledged that they were at a loss regarding how to teach them (Cronenwett et al., 2007). The QSEN Learning Collaborative was created to design strategies supporting quality and safety standards education. Representatives from diploma, AD, and BSN programs were chosen in relation to geographical location, school size, and faculty expertise in areas of classroom and clinical simulation. The group's goals included developing faculty expertise, promoting innovation in teaching, and introducing QSEN standards in textbooks, accreditation standards, and certification standards.

Since its inception, QSEN has had a significant impact on how nursing students are educated in schools around the country. Nursing faculty are assisting their students in obtaining the knowledge, skills, and attitudes that are increasingly important in ensuring safety cultures and reliable systems of care. In keeping with these goals, QSEN is incorporated throughout this text, showing the alignment of each standard with each chapter and its associated concepts and objectives.

The six QSEN standards provide guidance for nursing professionals to make the changes needed to create a safer, more effective health care delivery system. More importantly, QSEN teaches nurses to think differently and collaborate more efficiently, thus effecting positive change (Sherwood & Barnsteiner, 2012). As a valuable and realistic resource for everyone involved in the health care delivery system, QSEN provides better ways to secure safe and reliable health care.

Additionally, in order to reinforce the concepts presented in each chapter, associated ancillaries of case studies provided in an Instructor's Manual and PowerPoint presentation slides are available by email request to Springer Publishing Company: textbook@springerpub.com. I hope that students will find these exercises practical and useful in enhancing their knowledge.

The intent of this text is to celebrate and to welcome the LPN returning to school for a baccalaureate degree in nursing; to acknowledge what the LPN brings to the educational table; to introduce dynamic, current concepts in the nursing field; to scaffold new knowledge onto an existing solid nursing foundation; and to identify and realistically address students' recognized needs for a relatively seamless and successful transition to this new professional role.

REFLECTION EXERCISE

The intent of this text is to inspire you, spark interest in current endeavors in the profession, stimulate thought-provoking discussion among your colleagues, and provide practical, valuable evidence for use in your professional practice and continuing education.

Reflect on the following:

- How long have you been an LPN?
- Describe your LPN experience and current professional practice.

- Why did you decide to return to school? What made you choose this program?
- What strengths (personal and professional) do you feel you "bring to the table" in academia?
- What are your expectations about this course? This program? Achieving a baccalaureate degree in nursing?

Reflect on a personal story or anecdote that helps illustrate or reinforce your answers to the questions listed above.

Nancy Duphily

REFERENCES

Benner, P., Sutphen, M., Leonard, V., & Day, L. (2009). *Educating nurses: A call for radical transformation.* San Francisco, CA: Jossey-Bass.

Cronenwett, L., Sherwood, G., Barnsteiner, J., Disch, J., Johnson, J., Mitchell, P., . . . Warren, J. (2007). Quality and safety education for nurses. *Nursing Outlook, 55*(3), 122–131.

Dall'Alba, G. (2009). Learning professional ways of being: Ambiguities of becoming. *Educational Philosophy and Theory, 41*(1), 34–45.

Haas, J., & Shaffir, W. (1991). *Becoming doctors: The adoption of a cloak of competence.* Greenwich, CT: JAI.

Klossner, J. (2008). The role of legitimation in the professional socialization of second-year undergraduate athletic training students. *Journal of Athletic Training, 43*(4), 379–385.

Melrose, S., Miller, J., Gordon, K., & Janzen, K. (2012). Becoming socialized into a new professional role: LPN to BN student nurses' experiences with legitimation. *Nursing Research and Practice, 2012,* 1–8. ID 946063.

Sherwood, G., & Barnsteiner, J. (2012). *Quality and safety in nursing: A competency approach to improving outcomes.* Ames, IA: Wiley-Blackwell.

Spoelstra, S., & Robbins, L. (2010). A qualitative study of role transition from RN to APN. *International Journal of Nursing Education Scholarship, 7,* 20.

Acknowledgments

In writing this book, I am reminded of the significant contributions of those nursing students, nurses, and nurse educators who have given me the inspiration and incentive to pursue this venture.

I would like to thank the following people:

Present and former nursing students: Zachary Wright, for his contribution of an outstanding example of a nursing care plan; Roberta Farina, for her willingness to share her comprehensive client teaching plan; Jamy Gaynor, for providing a different perspective on teaching plans with her creative teaching/learning PowerPoint presentation; and Susan Provost, for supplying a quality concept map.

Donna Tully, nurse educator, for sharing her expertise with the development of a new and improved care plan template.

Elizabeth Nieginski, for her commitment to the idea and guidance throughout the project.

Nursing colleagues: educators, role models, mentors, and friends for life.

All of the nursing students, past and present, for sharing their stories.

PART I

Introduction to Role Transition

CHAPTER 1

The LPN/LVN and Baccalaureate Nursing Roles: Differences and Distinctions

OBJECTIVES

1. Analyze the change process.
2. Discuss Benner's stages of clinical competence.
3. Examine your philosophy of nursing.
4. Recognize the importance of performance evaluation and feedback.
5. Identify strategies to promote civility in nursing settings.
6. Describe stress reduction measures.

KEY TERMS

American Nursing
  Association (ANA)
  Standards of Practice

Change

Code of Ethics

Novice to expert

Nurse Practice Act

Performance evaluation

Philosophy of nursing

Refreezing

Stress

Transition

Unfreezing

STANDARDS

Teamwork and Collaboration		
Definition: Function effectively within nursing and interprofessional teams, fostering open communication, mutual respect, and shared decision making to achieve quality patient care.		
Knowledge	**Skills**	**Attitudes**
Describe own strengths, limitations, and values in functioning as a member of a team	Demonstrate awareness of own strengths and limitations as a team member. Initiate plan for self-development as a team member Act with integrity, consistency, and respect for differing views	Acknowledge own potential to contribute to effective team functioning. Appreciate importance of intra- and inter-professional collaboration
Describe scopes of practice and roles of health care team members. Describe strategies for identifying and managing overlaps in team member roles and accountabilities Recognize contributions of other individuals and groups in helping patient/family achieve health goals	Function competently within own scope of practice as a member of the health care team. Assume role of team member or leader based on the situation Initiate requests for help when appropriate to situation Clarify roles and accountabilities under conditions of potential overlap in team member functioning Integrate the contributions of others who play a role in helping patient/family achieve health goals	Value the perspectives and expertise of all health team members. Respect the centrality of the patient/family as core members of any health care team Respect the unique attributes that members bring to a team, including variations in professional orientations and accountabilities

(*continued*)

Knowledge	Skills	Attitudes
Analyze differences in communication-style preferences among patients and families, nurses, and other members of the health team. Describe impact of own communication style on others Discuss effective strategies for communicating and resolving conflict	Communicate with team members, adapting own style of communicating to needs of the team and situation. Demonstrate commitment to team goals Solicit input from other team members to improve individual, as well as team, performance Initiate actions to resolve conflict	Value teamwork and the relationships upon which it is based. Value different styles of communication used by patients, families, and health care providers Contribute to resolution of conflict and disagreement
Describe examples of the impact of team functioning on safety and quality of care. Explain how authority gradients influence teamwork and patient safety	Follow communication practices that minimize risks associated with handoffs among providers and across transitions in care. Assert own position/ perspective in discussions about patient care Choose communication styles that diminish the risks associated with authority gradients among team members	Appreciate the risks associated with handoffs among providers and across transitions in care
Identify system barriers and facilitators of effective team functioning. Examine strategies for improving systems to support team functioning	Participate in designing systems that support effective teamwork	Value the influence of system solutions in achieving effective team functioning

So never lose an opportunity of urging a practical beginning, however small, for it is wonderful how often in such matters the mustard-seed germinates and roots itself.

Florence Nightingale

TRANSITION: A PERSONAL STORY

I have always wanted to be a nurse. I always wanted to make someone feel better or save someone. I can honestly say that it was the best decision that I have ever made. I have always wanted to go back to school and further my education, but it was never a good time for me with working and raising small children. Now is the time.

Many positions require a bachelor's degree and it has also been said that some hospitals will only allow BSNs to work for them. Working in a Magnet Hospital, there is also a great push to further your education. As a member of the Practice Council at my job, I am surrounded by many overachievers, which can be intimidating. I want to be the best I can be as a professional for myself, the hospital, and for the benefits of my patients. I am hoping that gaining a baccalaureate degree in nursing will give me the skills to raise my level of critical thinking, communication, and teaching.

Nursing student

THE CHANGE PROCESS

Education is the most powerful weapon which you can use to change the world.

Nelson Mandela

Kurt Lewin developed his classic Change Theory in 1951, identifying three stages of change: **unfreezing, transition, and refreezing**. Lewin's theory is based on restraining and driving forces, creating a "push–pull" effect. Restraining forces are those life experiences that resist change (fears, threats), while driving forces provide incentive to change (personal goals, career advancement).

Unfreezing relates to a basic tendency of people to seek out an environment of relative safety in order to maintain a sense of control. In this way, they attach their sense of identity to their environment. This creates a comfortable stasis from which any alternatives, even those that may offer significant benefit, will cause discomfort. Talking about the future will not necessarily transfer them out of this "frozen" state. Substantial effort may be needed to "unfreeze" them and motivate them for readiness to change. Some individuals are "change ready," while others take time to leave their comfort zone.

Transition focuses on the belief that change is a journey rather than a simple step. Individuals may need to experience different stages of misunderstanding before they advance. A typical trap occurs when leaders spend time with their own personal journey, and then expect everyone else to "cross the chasm in a single bound." Transitioning is arduous and requires time and support. Quite often, the hardest part of this stage is to start. Individuals can become comfortable in temporary situations, where they are not accountable for the risks of work and where talking about change may be substituted for action.

The final goal, **refreezing,** involves putting down roots again and establishing a new place of stability. This stage is often rather uncertain, as a new change may well be around the next corner. This can lead to a state of "slush"; freezing is never attained. In this case, people fall into a state of "change shock," where they work at a low level of efficiency and effectiveness as they await the next change.

Transitioning and socialization are change processes. In pursuing a baccalaureate degree in nursing, LPNs may experience many interpersonal and intrapersonal emotions and conflicts along the way. In working through the change process from unfreezing to refreezing, LPNs are better equipped to successfully face and navigate these challenging "waters" during a nursing career of lifelong learning.

BENNER'S STAGES OF CLINICAL COMPETENCE

Patricia Benner (1984) incorporates the concepts of change, transition, and socialization in her iconic work, *From Novice to Expert*. Written not only for the individual entering nursing, but also for those in the profession who are seeking a new area of practice or additional education for advanced practice, Benner's research examines the acquisition of skills.

Within her own practice, Patricia Benner, RN, PhD, University of California School of Nursing, Department of Psychological Nursing (Benner, 1984), was concerned with how nurses acquire their nursing knowledge.

Following her nursing experience on an intensive care unit, Benner began researching the pathways by which individuals became nurses. Benner believed that experience within a profession, along with reflection upon that experience, assists nurses to develop their knowledge and to become experts in their individual field (Benner, Tanner, & Chesla, 2009).

Benner (1984) applied the Dreyfus Model of Skill Acquisition (Dreyfus & Dreyfus, 1980) when she published her research, *From Novice to Expert: Excellence and Power in Clinical Nursing Practice*. The accounts of experiences from practicing nurses enabled her to describe skill levels, in Stages 1 through 5, and articulate best-practice learning techniques for each level. Benner believes the most important way nurses can enhance their practice is through experience. The stages outlined are crucial for the nurse to transition from novice to expert roles.

During **Stage 1, the novice (beginner)** has no experience in the situations and expectations of performance. The novice requires repeated verbal and physical cues. Whether a beginner entering the profession or a veteran nurse changing specialties, the nurse will be expected to function in situations with no prior experience. With the experience gained from patient care, the novice develops the skills for working through actual situations.

In **Stage 2, the advanced beginner** demonstrates marginally acceptable performance from experience in actual situations. The nurse in Stage 2 is efficient and skillful in certain practice areas, yet needs periodic support and prompting. Advanced beginners have sufficient experience to be able to gather and interpret subjective and objective data. Advanced beginners rely on rules; however, with experience, they develop an awareness of additional characteristics that can be applied to related conditions.

Stage 3 describes the **competent nurse**, who has been employed in the same or similar settings for over 2 years. Competent nurses display efficiency, coordination, and confidence in their practice. They have become adept at planning, which aids efficiency and organization. Care is completed within a suitable time frame, without supporting cues. In planning care, the competent nurse incorporates both "conscious and abstract information" and "analytic contemplation of the situation" (Benner, 1984, p. 20). The outcome is enhanced efficiency, organization, and time management.

The **proficient nurse** of **Stage 4** has been employed in the same or similar settings for 3 to 5 years. In this stage, the proficient nurse considers situations in their entirety. With a holistic approach, proficient nurses anticipate which outcomes to expect in a particular situation, and are able to modify the plan of care, respond efficiently and effectively to events, and meet the individualized needs of patients. In this stage, the proficient nurse demonstrates skill in the ability to prioritize problems and to make informed decisions.

Within **Stage 5**, the **expert nurse** possesses an instinctive understanding of each situation and demonstrates the ability to focus directly on the core of a problem. Examining each situation from a holistic viewpoint, the expert nurse's performance is informed, efficient, and organized. Highly skilled analytic ability is critical for new situations encountered and prevents precious time and energy expended on other findings. Years of experience contribute to the expert nurse's intuitive grasp of the problem and skill in timely intervention.

Kaminski (2010) cites deliberate practice and a willingness to take risks as vital steps in successful evolution to the expert level. Deliberate practice involves a personal, goal-oriented approach to skill and knowledge development. Individuals experience personal satisfaction in confronting challenges to achieve a high standard of excellence within their field.

In risk taking, Kaminski states that progress through the novice to expert stages is not without challenges. However, the true expert must accept that the transition involves risks. Nurses will "continue to move up the ladder of skill and knowledge acquisition despite potential conflict within the nursing workplace" (Kaminski, 2010).

WHAT IS YOUR PHILOSOPHY OF NURSING?

As Kaminski (2010) cites, the move to a new area of nursing practice involves a certain amount of risk taking. Prior to transitioning to a new role or a return to academia, you may have given a considerable amount of thought to leaving the comfort zone of a job that for a period of time met your professional and personal needs. What brings nurses to take on new challenges?

Many nursing professionals find that changing demands and expectations of the role exceed the time and resources needed to carry out quality nursing care. Others cite the need for a new challenge and the opportunity to advance their practice. For these and other reasons, nurses are examining their current practice, their values, beliefs, and what attracted them to the profession in the first place.

A strategy to validate that one's nursing practice is consistent with one's value system is to write a personal philosophy statement. Doheny, Cook, and Stopper (1997) define philosophy as "beliefs of a person or group [of] persons . . . revealing underlying values and attitudes regarding an area" (p. 259). Philosophy looks at the nature of things with the intention of providing the meaning of phenomena. Nursing philosophy involves beliefs and principles about the nature of knowledge and truth, as well as about the nature of nursing practice and human healing processes.

Writing a personal philosophy statement first involves identification, clarification, and prioritization of our values. Our personal values are influenced by family, culture, religious orientation, education, and work. They influence our beliefs, actions, and who we are.

Included in a personal philosophy statement are values that relate to nursing. Concepts may come from the American Nurses Association (ANA) Code for Nurses and may incorporate ethics, professionalism, autonomy, accountability, caring, confidentiality, and integrity. The roles of caregiver, advocate, collaborator, educator, leader, and researcher may be considered for inclusion in the statement.

A personal philosophy statement should conclude with a summary of how personal values interrelate with values in nursing. Additional consideration should be given to incorporating strategies to achieve balance and professional growth through caring for oneself as well as others, through lifelong learning, and through emulating positive health promotion practices for the benefit of clients, colleagues, and loved ones.

COMMUNICATION AND PERFORMANCE EVALUATION: FEEDBACK

Along the lines of achieving personal health promotion practices, nurses must be able to seek out, accept, and act on the constructive feedback of others. In doing so, they can positively identify and address areas of growth. Accepting feedback is not always easy. In this process of "becoming" (Dall'Alba, 2009, p. 34) cited earlier in the preface to this book, nurses as lifelong learners are continually evaluated by others: clients, families, colleagues, supervisors, and various members of the health care team. We role model, mentor, problem solve, and teach others on a daily basis; these activities do not go unnoticed.

Asking for and receiving feedback require courage. Regardless of whether you choose to act on the information, it is important to know how you are perceived by others. Feedback is information we receive from others about the impact of our behavior on them. It allows us to view ourselves from another's perspective (Balzer-Riley, 2008).

The process of performance appraisal, usually performed annually, is a formal means of evaluating and providing feedback on your professional activities. When implemented appropriately, performance appraisal can be a highly effective tool for recognition and validation of outstanding work. Additionally, it provides motivation for the employee to continue this high-level performance and to strive for even greater accomplishments.

It is up to you, not your supervisor, to manage your career and to attain the level of recognition necessary for advancement. Nurse managers have multiple responsibilities and evaluate many employees under their supervision. Looking out for your career is not one of them. In preparation for your evaluation, it is important for you to maintain and bring to the meeting copies of your accomplishments, projects completed, plans for further education, and continuing education activities. Moreover, you should be prepared to discuss your professional goals for the upcoming year.

The main purpose of evaluation is to identify strengths and areas requiring attention, which will ultimately contribute to your professional growth. Motivation is the goal. Julia Balzer-Riley (2011) recommends the following steps during the evaluation process:

Focus: Listen carefully to what your evaluator is saying. Ensure that you are not distracted by other issues and can give your full attention to the information you are receiving.

Time: Allow sufficient time during the meeting in order to read through each point made on your evaluation, and reflect on the information without being rushed.

Understanding: Seek clarification or ask for repetition of feedback that is unclear.

Guidance: If the feedback indicates the need for a change in behavior, ask for advice or directions for change.

Appreciation: The evaluator providing feedback has taken the time and effort to provide you with useful information. Thank this individual for doing so.

Reflection: Evaluate your behavior in light of this new information. Reflect on the implications and consider changes.

If the evaluation is not what you expected, ask for more time to review the report and request another meeting to continue the discussion. This gives you the time to compose yourself and avoids an impulsive or defensive reaction, which can only undermine your standpoint. If you sign the evaluation, it is appropriate to write "signature reflects receipt of report only." You may attach a written response as well.

Following a second meeting, if you and your evaluator cannot come to an agreement over the evaluation, you can appeal the findings by consulting your employee handbook and/or by following the chain of command in your organization. At some point, you may have to decide how far the matter is worth pursuing. You may come to the realization that for your personal and professional health, it is best to leave the position or the organization.

COMMUNICATING TO PREVENT STRESS AND BURNOUT

Remaining in a position where conflict is the modus operandi in your organization and where one's daily stress level is consistently high is debilitating and, inevitably, severely compromises health. Nursing is demanding work, with long hours in high-stress environments caring for vulnerable clients. The decisions we make as nurses significantly impact the lives of clients.

Statistics demonstrate that rates of stress and burnout among nurses have been found to be higher than the rates among other health care professionals. Approximately 40% of hospital nurses have burnout levels higher than the norm for health care professionals (Aiken et al., 2001). Professional consequences of burnout have serious implications not only for nurses' health and well-being but also for the health and safety of clients. Moreover, fallout from stress and burnout reaches beyond the job itself and into the private lives of health care professionals. The emotional demands and other stressors in the health care environment break down emotional resources, with the potential for addictive behaviors (Office of Applied Studies, Substance Abuse and Mental Health Services Administration, 2008).

Numerous negative professional outcomes can be linked to prolonged stress and burnout, with poor work performance as the ultimate result. Emotional exhaustion leads to absenteeism and decreased productivity. The resultant fallout leads to work overload for nursing colleagues as well as client safety concerns. Nurses experiencing stress and burnout create distance between themselves and clients as well as colleagues. This depersonalization potentially decreases the quality of care, as cited by Maslach (2003) in *Burnout: The Cost of Caring*:

> Motivation is down, frustration is up, and an unsympathetic, don't-give-a damn attitude predominates. They don't take care in making their judgments, and they don't care as much about the outcome. They "go by the book" and are stale rather than innovative and fresh. They give the bare minimum rather than giving their all, and sometimes they give nothing at all. (p. 130)

So what steps can nurses take to avoid the downward spiral of stress, burnout, and ultimately compromised personal health?

COMMUNICATION: INCIVILITY IN THE NURSING PROFESSION

Scene 1: A veteran nurse rolls her eyes at the younger charge nurse who has created the morning assignment. Scene 2: A nurse on her way to the break room passes her coworker in the hallway. The coworker states she is overwhelmed by her heavy assignment. The nurse responds that she is "too busy" to help her out. Scene 3: A newly hired RN, formerly working as an LPN at the same hospital for over 10 years, finds he is now avoided by his colleagues.

While these scenarios may be labeled differently (lateral or horizontal violence, bullying, nurses "eating their young"), they are all prime examples of incivility. Clark and Ahten (2010) define incivility as "rude, disruptive, intimidating, and undesirable behaviors that are directed toward another person" (p. 9) and state that "uncivil behaviors affect recruitment and retention in the profession . . . students leave nursing programs, nurses leave the bedside, educators leave the classroom, and the profession suffers . . . ultimately, the public suffers too" (p. 10).

Incivility flourishes when individuals are stressed, overwhelmed, upset, and rushed. It can manifest overtly (name calling, fault finding, criticism, intimidation, gossip, shouting, blaming) or covertly (unfair assignments, avoidance, refusing to work with certain people or not work with others, whining, sabotage, exclusion, fabrication). Forni (2008) maintains that this behavior reduces one's self-esteem, ruins relationships, infects the work environment, and can often result in aggression and violence.

Estimates of lateral violence in the nursing workplace range from 46% to 100% (Stanley, Martin, Michel, Welton, & Nemeth, 2007). Johnson and

Rea (2009) reported that 27.3% of emergency department nurses experienced workplace incivility within a 6-month period. Staff described bullying behaviors by managers, charge nurses, nursing directors, physicians, and peers. Not unlike a virus, if tolerated from individuals with strong personalities, the behavior travels throughout the entire health care team, eventually reaching the client.

Gaps in nursing communication and the resultant disruption in teamwork are root causes of errors. When nurses fear retribution from intimidation, the client ultimately suffers. Research shows that simply witnessing rude behavior seriously affects the ability to execute cognitive tasks (Pearson & Porath, 2009). From an ethical perspective, tolerating bullying behaviors violates the nursing profession's pledge to keep clients safe (ANA, 2010).

Clark and Ahten (2010) advise the injured party to reflect on the experience before an impulsive response. In taking the time to calm down, the individual may choose not to respond at all. The authors support avoidance of poorly expressed messages, such as e-mail, hurried responses, or misperceptions of intent. Both individuals should agree on a mutually beneficial time and place to hold this critical conversation, in a venue that is quiet and will allow them to speak undisturbed. A third person can be invited by either side to mediate, if desired.

The selection of an appropriate meeting environment for this type of conversation is key. It should take place in a private area, away from patients, families, and other staff. Ideally, the organization should provide a safe, structured process for addressing the conflict, guaranteeing due process for all parties involved. The Joint Commission (2008) published a sentinel alert requiring all accredited health care organizations to implement codes of conduct and establish a formal process for managing unacceptable behavior.

Early on in the curriculum, nursing students should be educated regarding incivility in the profession. It does the new graduate/new employee a disservice to not have these experiences during their nursing education. The health care organization should incorporate elements of these experiences into orientation planning for newly hired nurses and continuing education for all nurses. Clark and Ahten (2010) describe a general orientation for students admitted into the nursing program. Students participate in a 90-minute workshop focusing on the importance of respectful behaviors, civility, and norms of behavior in the academic environment, including social media interactions. This provides the foundation for conversations about civility and professional behaviors that continues throughout their nursing program.

In a recent article in *American Nurse Today*, Lower (2012) provides strategies for nursing leaders to promote civility in their environments:

1. Examine your own behavior and how you contribute to civility or incivility.
2. Take a "temperature check" on your unit to see how staff treat one another.
3. Don't listen to or tolerate rumors and gossip.
4. Encourage staff not to jump to conclusions about the intent or motives of other staff, patients, or families.
5. Stop the blame game and encourage a solutions orientation to problems.
6. Encourage acts of kindness among staff.
7. Go out of your way to say thank you and promote this behavior in staff.
8. Look for common ground in dealing with conflict.
9. Encourage the practice of forgiveness.
10. Make it safe for staff to ask questions and discuss problems.

It is crucial to emphasize and reinforce organizational commitment to civility. Each organization should have a conflict resolution policy with specific procedures for conflict resolution. A well-written and properly enforced conflict resolution policy guarantees that due process will be followed for all parties involved.

The purpose in addressing incivility is to advocate for recognition, prevention, education, and intervention. All of these factors must be addressed to effect behavioral and organizational cultural change. In her diary, Anne Frank (1947) wrote "how wonderful it is that nobody need wait a single moment before starting to improve the world." As sound advice for nurse leaders to consider, this quote lends credence to the fact that small, initial steps to promote civil behavior can produce powerful results.

STRATEGIES FOR PREVENTION OF STRESS AND BURNOUT

In times of stress, I try emulating the nurse I aspire to be most like. I will sit and ask myself "what would 'Laura' do?" It is at that point the nurse who I admire the most, complete with all her wonderful attributes, comes fully to mind. Immediately I hear her gentle voice and recall her knowledgeable and kind ways. She is my guiding light, and following her as my role model definitely contributes to my personal success as she bridges the gap between what I was and what I want to be.

Nursing student

Stress management techniques and other interventions to ensure psychosocial well-being should be a priority for both individuals and institutions/organizations, with a goal of preventing stress and managing it while in its early stages. Attention to personal and professional lifestyle habits is essential for individuals to prevent and manage stress effectively.

Self-care needs have particular emphasis for health care professionals, as nurses have been taught to put the care of others ahead of themselves. Self-care is essential for energizing, restoring, and maintaining the physical and emotional stamina to manage stress (Maslach, 2003). Maintaining a healthy lifestyle is vital to avoiding the physical effects of stress. Individuals have effectively managed stress in a variety of ways, including yoga, relaxation techniques, music, art, reading, journaling, and sports.

Managing stress requires a high level of self-awareness. Staying in tune with the signs and symptoms of stress overload and burnout is a continuous process. Nurses should remain alert to their use of unhealthy coping mechanisms, such as excessive use of caffeine, alcohol, or prescription medication; overeating/undereating; smoking; inactivity; or social withdrawal. Such habits can be difficult to change, and individuals should focus on changing one behavior at a time and should seek help from professional counseling if necessary.

Time management is a common source of burnout among nurses. Extending far beyond techniques to use time efficiently, it relates to effectively managing the balance between personal and professional time. More time away from work has been the most common suggestion from health care professionals for reducing stress and preventing burnout (Carr, 2006).

A first step in creating a better work/life balance is to quantify the amount of time currently spent in each primary aspect of life (work, home, leisure, and vacation) and then determine priorities and assign preferred amounts of time for each aspect. Creating a "time budget" (Carr, 2006, p. 69) can help to prevent work life from overshadowing all other aspects of life, which can be harmful to self-esteem, self-identity, and overall well-being (Trinkoff, Geiger-Brown, Brady, Lipscomb, & Muntaner, 2006):

- Set strict boundaries between work and nonwork (not bringing work home).
- Remain emotionally present in each aspect of life.
- Take time to "recover" after a particularly difficult time at work.
- Engage in personal activities that require focus (such as sports, hobbies, or community volunteering).
- Stay clear about priorities.

Nursing colleagues are in a unique position to understand each other's professional needs and stressors. Social support from coworkers is particularly significant in times of change and uncertainty in the work environment. Collegial encouragement offers comfort, insight, rewards, humor, help, and escape (Raiger, 2005).

Maslach (2003) defines and describes the importance of "working smarter": setting realistic goals, doing things differently (when possible), not taking things personally, and taking time away. Setting realistic goals involves moving from abstract, idealistic goals to well-defined, specific goals, which can help individuals gain a better sense of accomplishment. Varying work routines can help avoid feelings of being in a rut and provide a sense of better control. Taking things less personally involves taking the emotion out of negative interactions, looking at conflict situations objectively, and, by doing so, reducing stress. Emotional involvement can also be decreased by not bringing client problems home.

Working smarter also means taking time away and organizing time more effectively. A typical response to work overload is to work longer or harder to help make the situation "get better" (Maslach, 2003). This approach inevitably leads to worsening stress and burnout. In addition, long stretches of work time and increased hours per day lead to fatigue and the potential for errors in care (Trinkoff et al., 2006).

Nurses are encouraged to take time away from work, even if only for a few minutes, to walk, rest, or other forms of exercise. This form of "recharging" leads to increased productivity more effectively than working continuously (Carr, 2006). Other time management techniques include scheduling a block of uninterrupted time (no phones, pagers, or e-mails) to complete paperwork more efficiently, creating "to do" lists to gain control over tasks, and working on refining organizational skills.

Supporting changes in the work environment can help nurses increase a sense of control. Assessing the potential for burnout and taking steps toward prevention is a process that begins with one person who assumes a leadership role in a group effort. The individual leader engages a group of colleagues to work with organizational leaders to heighten awareness of common stress factors within the organization and to address issues that compromise patient safety and quality of care.

The ANA encourages nurses to be familiar with its position statements designed to ensure the health and safety of nurses and patients: "Regardless of the number of hours worked, each registered nurse has an ethical responsibility to carefully consider her/his level of fatigue when deciding whether to accept any assignment extending beyond the regularly scheduled work day or week, including a mandatory or voluntary overtime assignment" (ANA, 2006).

Although nurses control their emotions, they are not immune to grief. A healthy response to loss is important for avoiding burnout. Instead of masking emotions, health care professionals must learn how to grieve (Carr, 2006). This involves accepting the reality of the loss, experiencing the pain of grief, adjusting to the absence, and moving on with life. Nurses can draw strength from colleagues and others by communicating sadness, frustration, and grief, and can find solace in discussing what they were able to achieve with their dying patients, such as the ability to help manage pain and other symptoms.

Maintaining positive relationships with colleagues, physicians, and patients is often challenging and requires strong communication skills. Nurses can decrease their vulnerability to stress by taking advantage of programs that strengthen their communication skills and help them to become more adept at handling difficult situations.

CHAPTER 1 REFLECTIVE QUESTIONS

1. Describe a change process in which you have been involved. What was your role? What were your restraining forces? What were your driving forces? Were others motivated/mobilized in this process? If so, how?

2. Think of a situation that you would like to change. Identify both restraining and driving forces. What could be done to make the change process occur?

3. As you transition from the LPN to RN role, is this change in your life happening because of an external force or an internal force? What stage of Lewin's Change Theory are you currently undergoing?

4. As you read the description of Benner's (1984) *From Novice to Expert* work, where, as an LPN returning to school for a baccalaureate degree in nursing, do you think you "fit"? Where would you place yourself within this five-stage model? Can you identify a similar process during your beginning practice as an LPN? Why/why not?

5. In writing a personal philosophy of nursing, incorporate the following questions:

   a. Introduction: Who are you? Where do you practice nursing?

   b. Define nursing: What is nursing? Why does nursing exist? Why do you practice nursing?

   c. Assumptions or underlying beliefs about: Nurses? Patients? Other health care providers? Communities?

   d. Define the major domains of nursing and provide examples: person, health, environment, nursing.

   e. Summary: How are the domains connected? What is your vision of nursing for the future? What are the challenges that you will face as a nurse? What are your goals for professional development?

CHAPTER 2

Theoretical Foundations of Nursing

OBJECTIVES

1. Describe nursing frameworks and nursing theories.
2. Compare and contrast the work of selected nursing theorists:
   a. Patricia Benner
   b. Virginia Henderson
   c. Imogene King
   d. Madeleine Leininger
   e. Betty Neuman
   f. Florence Nightingale
   g. Dorothea Orem
   h. Callista Roy
   i. Jean Watson
3. Discuss the relationship of theoretical frameworks to current practice.

KEY TERMS

Conceptual framework	Nursing frameworks
Environment	Nursing theories
Health	Nursing theorists
Metaparadigm	Person
Models	Phenomena
Nursing	

STANDARDS

Evidence-Based Practice (EBP)		
Definition: Integrate best current evidence with clinical expertise and patient/family preferences and values for delivery of optimal health care.		
Knowledge	Skills	Attitudes
Demonstrate knowledge of basic scientific methods and processes. Describe EBP to include the components of research evidence, clinical expertise, and patient/family values	Participate effectively in appropriate data collection and other research activities. Adhere to institutional review board (IRB) guidelines Base individualized care plan on patient values, clinical expertise, and evidence	Appreciate strengths and weaknesses of scientific bases for practice. Value the need for ethical conduct of research and quality improvement Value the concept of EBP as integral to determining best clinical practice
Differentiate clinical opinion from research and evidence summaries. Describe reliable sources for locating evidence reports and clinical practice guidelines	Read original research and evidence reports related to area of practice. Locate evidence reports related to clinical practice topics and guidelines	Appreciate the importance of regularly reading relevant professional journals
Explain the role of evidence in determining best clinical practice. Describe how the strength and relevance of available evidence influence the choice of interventions in provision of patient-centered care	Participate in structuring the work environment to facilitate integration of new evidence into standards of practice. Question rationale for routine approaches to care that result in less-than-desired outcomes or adverse events	Value the need for continuous improvement in clinical practice based on new knowledge

THEORY TO PRACTICE: NURSING STUDENTS' PERSPECTIVES

*What I find most impressive about Nightingale is that she equated envi-
ronment with health during a time when not much was developed in
terms of microbiology. Her health promotions were pure and simple, as
her practice applied to the rudimentary needs for good health and basic
survival as well. She was able to pinpoint the essentials of hygiene,
nutrition and healing without any previous role models to follow.*

 *Neuman's perspectives regarding stress can be applied to the
nurse as well, as we all know at times nursing can be quite stress-
ful. Neuman's theory emphasizes "appropriate actions in stress-related
situations," which can be an effective tool nurses apply to daily practice. Having deeper insight to the factors that contribute to stress, and
the reactions to stress, will help the nurse function properly as well as
contribute to a higher quality and standard of care.*

Nursing student

*Mutual respect and a true sharing of both power and control are essential
elements of collaboration.*

Virginia Henderson (1991)

In the application of theory to practice, the nurse must possess an understanding of the theoretical frameworks from the nursing profession. This
chapter provides an introductory overview of selected works for further
reflection and study. You are encouraged to read more in-depth discussions
on nursing theoretical frameworks, starting with the references cited in this
chapter.

NURSING FRAMEWORKS AND NURSING THEORIES

For years, nursing has incorporated theories from other disciplines, including theories of systems, human needs, change, problem solving, and decision making. The profession's focus has changed significantly, from one
of only carrying out skills and tasks, to incorporating a basis in theory.
Application of theory to practice lends itself to increased depth and understanding of the role and the image of a professional nurse, and how the
nurse should care for clients.

 Nursing theories endeavor to describe or explain the phenomenon
of nursing (Barnum, 1998; Chinn & Jacobs, 1987). Incorporated into

these theories are concepts, definitions, relationships, and assumptions taken from nursing models, frameworks, and other disciplines. They portray a purposeful and organized viewpoint of phenomena by creating interrelationships among concepts to describe, explain, predict, and prescribe. In this way, nursing theory builds professional nursing practice, produces further knowledge, and directs future nursing practice.

Within nursing theories, four major concepts are integrated, which define and explain the discipline: **person, environment, health,** and **nursing. Persons** are the recipients of nursing care; this includes individuals, families, communities, and groups. **Environment** incorporates factors that affect individuals internally and externally, not only in everyday surroundings, but in all settings where nursing care is provided. **Health** generally addresses the person's state of well-being, while the concept of **nursing** is central to all nursing theories.

The following section presents a selection of influential nursing theorists who have helped to create and shape the present views on health, healing, and, ultimately, the professional practice of many nurses.

NURSING THEORISTS

Patricia Benner

Patricia Benner's nursing philosophy was first described in her book, *From Novice to Expert: Excellence and Power in Clinical Nursing Practice.* Benner provided examples of nursing practice based on observation and interviews with professionals ranging from those just starting their professional careers to veteran nurses. Her work demonstrated that clinical nursing practice was more complex than theories of nursing could describe, explain, or predict.

Benner used the Dreyfus Model of Skill Acquisition (Benner, 2004), which describes five levels of skill acquisition and development: novice, advanced beginner, competent, proficient, and expert. Her nursing philosophy describes growth and development in four areas as a nurse gains knowledge through experience. The first area concerns the ability to move from using abstract principles and rules to using past, concrete experiences. The second change demonstrates a shift from rule-based thinking to using intuition. The nurse who has acquired more clinical skill is increasingly able to see a patient situation as a complex whole, with some characteristics being more relevant than others. Lastly, the nurse becomes highly involved in the clinical situation.

Benner also described several domains of nursing practice, including the helping role, the teaching–coaching function, the diagnosis and patient monitoring function, effective management of rapidly changing situations, administering and monitoring therapeutic interventions, monitoring and ensuring the quality of health care practices, and organizational and work-role competencies. As nurses move on a developmental continuum from novice to expert, they are more able to excel in these nursing role domains.

Virginia Henderson

Contemporary nursing theory began with Virginia Henderson (1897–1996) in the 1960s. She developed a nursing model based on activities of living. Often regarded as "The Twentieth Century Florence Nightingale," Henderson defined nursing as "assisting individuals to gain independence in the performance of activities contributing to health or its recovery" (Henderson, 1966, p. 3). Henderson viewed nursing as apart from medicine; nursing was more than simply following the physician's orders. Henderson described nursing in relation to the client and the client's environment. Moreover, she advocated that teaching and advocacy roles were paramount to the profession. Her Needs Theory classified nursing activities into 14 components, grounded on human needs, a central focus of nursing practice. Further development of human needs is seen in later theories regarding the needs of the person and how nursing can assist in meeting those needs (Halloran & Thorson, 1996).

Henderson's emphasis on the importance of nursing's independence from and interdependence with other health care disciplines is well recognized (Blais & Hayes, 2011). Henderson's theory is current and applicable to professional nursing today. Nurses function to assist patients in activities of daily living, especially those who are incapable of doing so because of a debilitating condition.

Henderson defined nursing in functional terms: "The unique function of the nurse is to assist the individual, sick or well, in the performance of those activities contributing to health or its recovery (or to a peaceful death) that he would perform unaided if he had the necessary strength, will or knowledge . . . and to do this in such a way as to help him gain independence as rapidly as possible" (Tomey & Alligood, 1998, p. 102).

Imogene King

The basis for Imogene King's Theory of Goal Attainment (1960) is that the nurse and the patient communicate information, set goals together, and then take actions to achieve those goals. The Goal Attainment Theory defines an interpersonal relationship that encourages the individual to grow and develop in order to successfully achieve life goals (Lavin & Killeen, 2008).

King's theory is based on the following assumptions: Nursing's focus is the care of human beings; nursing's goal is the health care of individuals; human beings are open systems, interacting constantly with their environment; nurse and client communicate information, set goals mutually, and act to attain those goals; each human being perceives the world as a total person in making transactions with individuals and things in the environment; transaction represents a life situation in which the perceiver and the thing perceived are encountered; and a person enters the situation as an active participant and is changed in the process of these experiences (Frey, Sieloff, & Norris, 2002).

With the Goal Attainment Theory, the main function of nursing is to increase or to restore the health of the client. Transactions should occur to set goals related to the health of the client. After transactions have occurred and goals have been defined by the nurse and client together, both parties work toward the stated goals. This may involve interactions with other systems, such as other health care workers, the client's family, or larger systems.

Madeleine Leininger

Madeleine Leininger's Theory of Transcultural Care Diversity and Universality originates from anthropology and nursing. Leininger, an RN and a PhD in cultural and social anthropology, believed that care was the central aspect to nursing. Leininger viewed transcultural nursing as an area of study focused on cultural care values, beliefs, and practices of individuals of different cultures (Sitzman & Eichelberger, 2010).

With her theory rooted in clinical nursing practice, Leininger noted that clients from diverse cultures valued care more than nurses did. She determined that there existed a need to develop a theoretical framework to discover, explain, and predict dimensions of care. From the outcome of her studies conducted in numerous Western and non-Western cultures, Leininger developed the Culture Care Diversity and Universality Theory, depicted as the "Sunrise Enabler" (George, 2011, p. 410).

The wide variety of existing cultures in society today presents challenges in order to best meet the health care needs of the diverse client. "The goal . . . is to provide culture-specific, universal nursing care practices in promoting health or well-being . . . or to help people to face

unfavorable human conditions, illness, or death in culturally meaningful ways" (Sitzman & Eichelberger, 2011). Nurses cannot properly care
for clients if they cannot know them or understand their needs. Caring
is essential to curing and healing; there can be no curing without caring.
Clients who experience nursing care contradictory to their beliefs and
values will exhibit signs of cultural conflict, noncompliance, and stress.
Leininger believes that "the qualitative paradigm provides ways of knowing and discovering the epistemic and ontological dimensions of human
care transculturally" (Leininger, 1991, p. 45).

Key concepts in this theory include cultural diversity (the differences
between and among different cultures) and cultural universality (commonali-
ties or similarities in different cultures). With Leininger's theory, nurses can
recognize and understand those cultural similarities and differences that influence the individual's health status. In an era of globalization, coupled with an
increasing emphasis on cultural awareness to meet the needs of a diverse client population, Leininger's theory is particularly current and relevant.

Betty Neuman

In Betty Neuman's Systems Model (NSM), the individual is viewed as an
open system interacting with both internal and external environment forces
and stressors. Continuously changing, individuals move toward a dynamic
state of system stability, or toward states of illness, in varying degrees. In
the NSM, nursing is considered a system; nursing practice involves components of the system that interact with each other. Within the system, there is
a continuous diversity of nursing roles and functions (George, 2011).

Client variables are physiological, psychological, sociocultural, developmental, and spiritual stressors (Neuman & Fawcett, 2011). The client system
consists of a core structure protected by lines of resistance. The usual level
of health is a normal line of defense that is protected by a flexible line of
defense. Stressors are intra-, inter-, and extra-personal in nature, developing
from internal, external, and created environments. When stressors invade
the flexible line of defense, the lines of resistance are activated. If adequate
energy exists, the system will be rebuilt and the lines of defense restored
(Neuman, 2001).

Nursing interventions take place at three areas of prevention: primary prevention, that is, before the stressor invades the system; secondary prevention, after the system reacts to an invading stressor; and tertiary
prevention, after secondary prevention as reconstitution is established.

Health is defined as the condition or degree of system stability and is considered on a wellness-to-illness scale. When system needs are met, optimum wellness exists. When needs are not satisfied, illness exists. When the necessary energy needed to support life is unavailable, death occurs (DeWan & Ume-Nwagbo, 2006).

The primary concern of nursing is to define the appropriate action in situations that are stress-related, or related to client/client-system responses to stressors. Nursing interventions are designed to help the system adapt and to return and/or preserve stability between "the client system variables and environmental stressors" with a focus on conserving energy (George, 2011, p. 354).

Florence Nightingale

Florence Nightingale, the "Lady with the Lamp," is considered to be the founder of modern nursing. Raised in a wealthy family where women were not allowed to work, it was against her family's wishes when she decided to pursue nursing. At 31, Nightingale traveled to the Deaconess Institute in Kaiserswerth, Germany, where she trained for 3 months. During the Crimean War of 1854 to 1856, Nightingale's care of the soldiers became legendary. Nightingale found the conditions in the army hospital in Scutari appalling. The men were without blankets or decent food. War wounds accounted for only one death in six; typhus, cholera, and dysentery were responsible for the high death rates among wounded soldiers.

Following the war, Nightingale continued to carry out her nursing work despite limitations acquired from Crimean sickness, which kept her bedridden for the remainder of her life. From her bed, she wrote daily. From the meticulous statistics she maintained during the Crimean War, Nightingale was responsible for helping to reform the military medical record-keeping system.

In 1859, she authored her famous *Notes on Nursing* (MacQueen, 2007), which expanded on the definition of nursing and introduced the Environmental Theory. This model promoted the importance of ventilation and warming, noise reduction, adequate lighting, appropriate bedding, personal cleanliness, and proper nutrition (MacQueen, 2007). A central theme concerned nursing's role in the management of the patient environment (Selander & Crane, 2012). The conditions at Scutari reinforced her viewpoint, and led to her advocacy for the importance of an appropriate environment for the patient, both internally and externally.

Nightingale's lasting legacy is a blending of her many accomplishments and her vision of what can and should be undertaken by the profession. Her legendary accomplishments have become the "roadmap for future generations" (Selander & Crane, 2012).

Dorothea Orem

Dorothea Orem is well known for her Self-Care Nursing Deficit Theory, also recognized as the Orem Theory of Nursing, which supports health promotion and health maintenance. Self-care implies that when they are able, individuals care for themselves. When the person is unable to do so, the nurse provides the assistance needed. As a liaison, the nurse's role is to promote the client's ability for self-care through education and direct, individualized nursing care. The nurse and client work as a team to achieve self-care. The nurse also maintains a collaborative approach with other members of the health care team to provide consistent, continuous quality care. To promote healing through independence, the nurse supplies the client with the educational tools needed for successful achievement of this goal (Orem, 2001).

Orem's theory is composed of three interconnected theories: self-care, self-care deficit, and nursing systems. Within these theories are six central concepts of self-care, self-care agency, therapeutic care demand, self-care deficit, nursing agency, and nursing system. Nursing is needed when self-care demands are greater than self-care abilities. In determining the type of care needed, the nurse selects from among wholly compensatory, partly compensatory, and supportive–educative systems (George, 2011).

Consideration of the individual patient's needs is supported by Orem's theory and routinely applied within daily nursing practices. The theory advocates for nurses' recognition of different levels of understanding, cultures, and family dynamics. Ultimately, individualizing patients' needs leads to better understanding and improved client outcomes. As the client regains the ability to engage in self-care activities, the nurse functions in a supportive–educative mode.

Callista Roy

Sister Callista Roy's Adaptation Model (RAM) views a person as comprising interrelated biological, psychological, and social systems (Sitzman & Eichelberger, 2011). The four major concepts of the RAM are: "humans as adaptive systems as both individuals and groups; the environment; health; and the goal of nursing" (Roy & Andrews, 1999, p. 35). The model presents concepts related to these four areas, clarifying each and defining their interrelationships.

The individual (person) continuously seeks to maintain a balance among these systems as well as the external environment. The person is an open, adaptive system that employs coping skills to confront stressors. The goal of nursing is to promote the person's adaptation during health and illness using four adaptation modes: the physiological mode, the self-concept mode, the role function mode, and the interdependence mode (George, 2011).

The physiological mode deals with the maintenance of the physical body. This includes basic human needs such as air, water, food, and temperature regulation. The function of the mode of self-concept is the need for the maintenance of the mind. The person's perceptions of the physical and personal self are included in this mode. Social integrity is emphasized in the role function mode. This addresses people's adaptations to different role changes that occur throughout a lifetime. The interdependence mode also addresses social integrity, but deals with the balance between independence and interdependence in relationships with other people.

In Roy's model, health is defined as being or becoming an integrated whole person. The goal of nursing is to promote adaptation of the client during health and illness in all four of the modes. The nurse's actions begin with assessment on two levels: First, the nurse makes a judgment regarding the presence or absence of maladaptation; second, the nurse focuses on the stimuli influencing the client's behavior. At this point, the nurse acts to promote adaptation by manipulating the environment, components of the client system, or both as part of the nursing care plan.

The model proposes that nurses alter, increase, decrease, remove, or maintain the focal stimulus. If that is not possible, nurses may change the particular stimuli to support adaptation and transformation between the person and the environment (Roy & Andrews, 1999).

Jean Watson

Health as harmony within body, mind, and soul and the degree of convergence between self as perceived and self as experienced, determining health or illness, drive the goals of care in Watson's theory. The main conceptual elements of Watson's original Theory of Transpersonal Caring were the transpersonal caring relationship, the 10 carative factors, and caring occasion/caring moment. The evolving nature of Watson's theory led to the redefining and renaming of the original factors to 10 clinical Caritas Processes (Watson, 2005):

1. Embrace altruistic values and practice loving kindness with self and others.
2. Instill faith and hope and honor others.
3. Be sensitive to self and others by nurturing individual beliefs and practices.
4. Develop helping, trusting, caring relationships.
5. Promote and accept positive and negative feelings as you authentically listen to another's story.
6. Use creative scientific problem-solving methods for caring decision making.
7. Share teaching and learning that address the individual's needs and comprehension styles.
8. Create a healing environment for the physical and spiritual self that respects human dignity.
9. Assist with basic physical, emotional, and spiritual human needs.
10. Be open to mystery and allow miracles to enter.

The essence of Watson's theory is caring for the purpose of promoting healing, preserving dignity, and respecting the wholeness and interconnectedness of humanity. Her work characterizes nursing as a healing art and science devoted to the pursuit of harmonious and sacred relationships. Watson views each person as a human being to be valued, cared for, respected, nurtured, understood, and assisted within his or her environment (Cara, 2003).

Displaying factors of caring will help nurses feel a sense of job satisfaction. By practicing caring, nurses can ease patients' suffering. In this way, nurses instill a sense of hope and faith, which promotes healing. "Nursing can expand its existing role, continuing to make contributions to health care within the modern model by developing its foundational caring–healing and health strengths that have always been present on the margin" (Watson, 1999, p. 45).

Watson's theory emphasizes the humanistic aspects of nursing in combination with scientific knowledge. The theory was created to bring meaning and focus to nursing as a distinct health profession: "Caring is an endorsement of professional nurses' identity" (Watson, 2008). This statement is supported in Nightingale's work: "It is the surgeon who saves a person's life . . . it is the nurse who helps this person live."

SUMMARY

How does theory impact nursing practice? Using a theoretical framework to guide nursing practice assists the nurse to organize, understand, and analyze data, plan, carry out nursing interventions, and evaluate outcomes of care. As adjuncts to critical thinking when planning and providing nursing care, theoretical frameworks provide an efficient, educated approach to nursing practice.

Future challenges in the nursing profession involve making theory-based practice a reality. To be considered professionals, nurses must be able to define, describe, and educate others about the unique discipline of nursing. Theory provides a meaningful tool to articulate our message.

CHAPTER 2 REFLECTIVE QUESTIONS

Reflect on the work of the selected nursing theorists. Which theorist/theory do you feel is most closely aligned with your nursing practice, with your beliefs as a nurse? To assist you in your response, consider the following questions:

1. Why did I become a nurse?
2. What values and beliefs keep me in nursing?
3. What values about humans and nursing are most important to me?
4. How do I describe what nursing is and what nurses do to my family and friends?
5. Does a specific theory reflect nursing practice in a way that I value?
6. Will a specific theory support my concept of excellent nursing practice?
7. Which theories are most relevant to my practice area?
8. Can the theory help me explain, design, and evaluate care?

Professionalism in Nursing

OBJECTIVES

Describe and discuss the implications of the following:

1. American Nurses Association Standards of Care
2. Institute of Medicine Report/Recommendations
3. Carnegie Report (2010)
4. Quality and Safety Education for Nurses (QSEN) competencies
5. Nurse of the Future (NOF): Nursing Core Competencies
6. *The Essentials of Baccalaureate Education for Professional Nursing Practice*
7. American Association of Colleges of Nursing (AACN)
8. Nursing shortage
9. Advanced practice

KEY TERMS

Advanced practice

American Association of Colleges of Nursing (AACN)

American Nurses Association (ANA) Standards of Care

Baccalaureate Essentials

Carnegie Report

Commission on Collegiate Nursing Education (CCNE)

Institute of Medicine (IOM)

Nurse of the Future (NOF) Initiative

Nursing shortage

Quality and Safety Education for Nurses (QSEN)

STANDARDS

Teamwork and Collaboration		
Definition: Function effectively within nursing and interprofessional teams, fostering open communication, mutual respect, and shared decision making to achieve quality patient care.		
Knowledge	**Skills**	**Attitudes**
Describe own strengths, limitations, and values in functioning as a member of a team	Demonstrate awareness of own strengths and limitations as a team member. Initiate plan for self-development as a team member Act with integrity, consistency, and respect for differing views	Acknowledge own potential to contribute to effective team functioning. Appreciate importance of intra- and inter-professional collaboration
Describe scopes of practice and roles of health care team members. Describe strategies for identifying and managing overlaps in team member roles and accountabilities Recognize contributions of other individuals and groups in helping patient/family achieve health goals	Function competently within own scope of practice as a member of the health care team. Assume role of team member or leader based on the situation Initiate requests for help when appropriate to situation Clarify roles and accountabilities under conditions of potential overlap in team member functioning Integrate the contributions of others who play a role in helping patient/family achieve health goals	Value the perspectives and expertise of all health team members. Respect the centrality of the patient/family as core members of any health care team Respect the unique attributes that members bring to a team, including variations in professional orientations and accountabilities

(continued)

Knowledge	Skills	Attitudes
Analyze differences in communication-style preferences among patients and families, nurses, and other members of the health team. Describe impact of own communication style on others Discuss effective strategies for communicating and resolving conflict	Communicate with team members, adapting own style of communicating to needs of the team and situation. Demonstrate commitment to team goals Solicit input from other team members to improve individual, as well as team, performance Initiate actions to resolve conflict	Value teamwork and the relationships upon which it is based. Value different styles of communication used by patients, families, and health care providers Contribute to resolution of conflict and disagreement
Describe examples of the impact of team functioning on safety and quality of care. Explain how authority gradients influence teamwork and patient safety	Follow communication practices that minimize risks associated with handoffs among providers and across transitions in care. Assert own position/perspective in discussions about patient care Choose communication styles that diminish the risks associated with authority gradients among team members	Appreciate the risks associated with handoffs among providers and across transitions in care
Identify system barriers and facilitators of effective team functioning. Examine strategies for improving systems to support team functioning	Participate in designing systems that support effective teamwork	Value the influence of system solutions in achieving effective team functioning

A PERSONAL DEFINITION OF PROFESSIONALISM

I believe professionalism is a standard that a person holds themselves to, to deliver quality and proficient services to their clients…mastering a certain skill set that can be offered as a service. Professionalism is a confidence, poise, and knowledge that an individual possesses while rendering services. I also think professionalism is putting the job first and enhancing the work you do with your individual personality while never losing autonomy.

Nursing student

In my maternity clinical experience, I was assigned a 23-year-old homeless client, MM. When I met MM she was 1 day post C-section and appeared very sad and depressed. This young woman had her first child in high school at the age of 17 and the child had been placed in foster care 1 year later. MM had previously lived with her mother, a single parent with a history of alcoholism, but left at the age of 18 to stay with a friend. After a disagreement, MM was asked to leave the friend's apartment, and became homeless when her mother refused to let her move back in. With no other family in the area, MM had been living on the streets and moving between different shelters in the area when she became pregnant. I made it a point to check in on her regularly. As she shared the details of her life, it was apparent that MM had numerous social, economic, and emotional needs beyond [those] required by the typical new mother. The initial concern was her emotional state and the fact that she had nowhere to go upon discharge. The nurses were supportive, nonjudgmental, and professional in all aspects of MM's care. They encouraged MM to attend breastfeeding and bath demo classes offered by the hospital. While at first MM was skeptical about attending, she fully participated and was happy to have me accompany her there to share the experience.

I was also able to spend time with the nursing case manager as she worked to obtain services for MM. She, too, communicated with the client in a manner that was professional, appropriate, and sensitive to MM's situation, and thus received a positive reaction from the young woman. The nurses showed tremendous understanding and empathy toward MM, and they used effective communication skills to encourage her to bond with her baby. Transitional housing and nursing services for MM were arranged upon discharge. The entire nursing team made me proud to know that this was the profession I had chosen to pursue.

Nursing student

The following overview standards, initiatives, organizations, and reports are presented to inform the student returning to academia about significant issues that have shaped current practice and trends in the nursing profession. The reader is encouraged to take advantage of the information provided within the text for further explanation and discussion of each resource.

AMERICAN NURSES ASSOCIATION (ANA) STANDARDS OF NURSING CARE

Our lives begin to end the day we become silent about things that matter.

Martin Luther King, Jr.

A standard is a model of recognized practice that is generally accepted as true. Creating and applying standards of practice are key responsibilities of a professional organization. In professional nursing practice, standards of care (SOCs) refer to a competent level of nursing care. Developed by clinicians, administrators, and academic experts, the ANA Standards of Nursing Care guide the knowledge, skills, judgment, and attitudes crucial for safe nursing practice. Standards of nursing practice represent the beliefs and concerns of the profession and provide a framework for the evaluation of nursing practice. Standards outline nursing's accountability to the public (ANA, 2004).

According to the standards of care, a licensed nurse reports and documents nursing assessments or observations, the care provided to the client, and the client's response to that care. Nurses assume a liability risk if they fail to monitor, recognize, or communicate changes in a client's condition promptly to the attending practitioner. A nurse who cannot fulfill the accepted standards of care may be accused of negligence. Most legal actions against nurses arise when a client claims the nurse breached an SOC and that the breach resulted in harm to the client (McMahon, 2012). Malpractice (negligence on the part of a health care professional) is one legal action with which a nurse may be charged for failing to meet the SOC.

Nursing standards clearly reflect the specific functions and activities that nurses provide. The ANA's Nursing Scope and Standards of Practice consists of both standards of care and standards of professional performance. Standards of professional performance describe a "competent level of nursing and performance common to all registered nurses" (ANA, 2004, p. 1). The six standards of practice reflect the critical thinking model known as the nursing process and form the foundation for the nurse's decision making. The nine standards of professional performance describe competent behaviors in performing the nursing role. More information on the American Nurses Association (ANA) Standards of Care can be found at www.nursingworld.org/nursingstandards.

INSTITUTE OF MEDICINE (IOM) REPORT

This report is really about the future of health care in our country. It points out that nurses are going to have a critical role in that future, especially in producing safe, quality care and coverage for all patients in our health care system.

> Donna E. Shalala, PhD, Chair of the Committee of
> the Robert Wood Johnson Foundation Initiative
> on the Future of Nursing, at the IOM

In 2003, the IOM issued *Health Professions Education: A Bridge to Quality* (IOM, 2003). Focusing on the knowledge level required by health care professionals to provide quality care, the findings revealed that students in the health professions were unprepared to meet the country's current demographic shift. Moreover, students were unable to access evidence for use in practice, determine the reasons for client care errors, and access technology to acquire the latest information. The report expressed concern with the adequacy of nursing education at all levels and identified five core competencies clinicians should possess: provide patient-centered care; work in interdisciplinary teams; use evidence-based practice (EBP); apply quality improvement (QI) and identify errors and hazards in care; and utilize informatics (IOM, 2003).

In 2008, the Robert Wood Johnson Foundation (RWJF) and IOM responded to the challenge of assessing and transforming the nursing profession. The committee made the following four recommendations:

- Nurses should practice to the full extent of their education and training.
- Nurses should achieve higher levels of education and training through an improved education system that promotes seamless academic progression.

▥ Nurses should be full partners, with physicians and other health care professionals, in redesigning health care in the United States.

▥ Effective workforce planning and policy making require better data collection and information infrastructure.

Another study by the IOM (2010), *The Future of Nursing: Leading Change, Advancing Health,* explored nursing graduates' preparedness for practice in light of the changes and complexity of current practice and practice environments. The report challenges nursing education to construct major reforms in the preparation of new graduates. This involves establishing new competencies and outcomes for graduates, new curriculum designs, better evaluation models, and new models for clinical education, such as internships and residency programs. More information on the 2010 IOM report can be found at www.iom.edu/Reports/2010/The-future-of-nursing.

THE CARNEGIE REPORT

In *Educating Nurses: A Call for Radical Transformation*, authors Benner, Sutphen, Leonard, and Day (2011) outline their recommendations for restructuring nursing education to meet current and future needs of patients. The Carnegie Foundation National Nursing Education Study presents information from site visits to nursing programs, interviews, observations, and surveys of faculty and students.

The research team visited geographically and academically diverse schools, including a community college, a private liberal arts college, and a graduate-level state university focused exclusively on the health care professions. The team observed classes and interviewed administrators, faculty, and staff. Students were observed in the classroom, and in clinical, skills, and simulation laboratory settings.

An additional phase of the research study involved conducting a national survey of faculty and students. From the survey findings, the authors pointed out the challenges for educators to discover more effective approaches to teaching nursing, to help students apply knowledge effectively in practice, and to develop ethical conduct in teaching/learning settings (Benner et al., 2009). Teaching for intervention in client situations, integration of classroom and clinical teaching, and clinical reasoning were cited as additional tasks for educators.

The authors reported that nurses are undereducated for the demands of practice. Current nurse administrators are concerned with the practice-education gap, as it becomes more difficult for nursing education to keep up with the rapid changes in research and technology. Their recommendations stress the following: advocating for the baccalaureate degree in entry-level nursing practice; increasing the number of second-degree baccalaureate and master's programs; requiring a postgraduate year of internship in a clinical setting; recruiting a diverse faculty and student population that reflects the health care population served; providing more financial aid for students; and maintaining clinical postconferences and manageable patient care assignments (Benner et al., 2009).

Educators should use both formative and summative assessments, including simulation exercises, skills laboratories, classrooms with actor patients, and assessments done directly in the clinical setting. Indicators of clinical performance should include how well students are able to set priorities in particular clinical situations, develop rationales for patient care, and respond to changes in patients. Students should also be assessed on their skills of clinical reasoning and their ability to solve clinical puzzles (Vitello-Cicciu, 2010).

Transformation in nursing practice requires corresponding changes in both the education of nurses and the preparation of nurse educators. The challenge will be to create health care organizations that will educate nurses in a climate that encourages professional focus, accountability, and quality (Vitello-Cicciu, 2010). More information on the Carnegie Report can be found at www.carnegiefoundation.org/nursing-education.

QUALITY AND SAFETY EDUCATION FOR NURSES (QSEN)

Nursing practice based on evidence is now the recognized standard for practice as well as one of the six core competencies identified in the QSEN project (Cronenwett et al., 2007, 2009).

The 1999 study conducted by the IOM, *To Err Is Human: Building a Safer Health System,* revealed that the estimated annual cost of medical errors in hospitals across the country ranged from $17 billion to $29 billion at hospitals, with resultant death rates between 44,000 and 98,000 (IOM, 1999). The report prompted The Joint Commission and the Agency for Healthcare Research and Quality (AHRQ, n.d.) to act by developing standards for health care organizations to reduce the number of errors.

In 2005, the RWJF funded a national study to educate nurses about client safety and quality. A three-tiered plan was created to address the education–practice gap: In Phase I, a team of experts examined factors related to quality and safety; Phase II involved the development of QSEN competencies; and

Phase III focused on integration of the competencies into curricula, research, accreditation, and licensing. The overall goal was to improve client outcomes by providing nursing students with the knowledge, skills, and attitudes needed to provide safe and effective quality care (Hunt, 2012).

QSEN's initiative is directed to develop competencies of future nursing graduates in six key areas: client-centered care; teamwork and collaboration; EBP; QI; safety; and informatics. For each competency, expectations relating to knowledge (understanding), skills (implementation), and attitudes (values) must be attained. Nursing graduates should have achieved these competencies and transferred them over to their professional practice role.

The first competency, patient-centered care, focuses on including patients in all decisions and providing compassionate care based on needs and values. The second competency, teamwork and collaboration, relates to shared decision making among health care team members. The third competency, EBP, involves using current evidence when providing care. The fourth competency, QI, incorporates data collection, evaluation, and improvement of patient outcomes. Safety, the fifth competency, centers on preventing harm to patients. Informatics is the basis for the sixth competency, that is, the application of technology to promote safety and quality. Technology is always improving, and the use of electronic medical records (EMRs), medication administration programs, and other equipment and programs has been shown to improve patient safety.

Although many of the QSEN competencies are part of health care settings, nurses are encouraged to continue to integrate them into practice. The overall goal of the QSEN project is to meet the challenge of preparing future nurses who will have the knowledge, skills, and attitudes necessary to continuously improve the quality and safety of the health care systems within which they work.

The QSEN competencies can be found at http://qsen.org/about-qsen.

NURSE OF THE FUTURE (NOF) INITIATIVE

The NOF project agenda was created at a 2-day working session sponsored by the Department of Higher Education (DHE) and the Massachusetts Organization of Nurse Executives (MONE) in 2006. Attended by statewide stakeholders in nursing education and practice, the group reviewed standards, initiatives, and best practices in nursing education. The Massachusetts NOF Competency Committee was responsible for identifying a core set of nursing competencies; the MONE Academic Practice Integration Committee was charged with using the identified competencies as a framework for developing a statewide transition into practice model. A steering committee was also ultimately created to oversee approaches toward completing the priorities and setting the ongoing agenda. From this assembly, members created the Nurse of the Future: Nursing Core Competencies (Massachusetts Department of Higher Education [MDHE], 2010). This document addresses the knowledge base and relationships among concepts important to nursing practice. The 10 Nurse of the Future Core Competencies are as follows:

1. Patient-centered care
2. Professionalism
3. Leadership
4. Systems-based practice
5. Informatics and technology
6. Communication
7. Teamwork and collaboration
8. Safety
9. QI
10. EBP

The committee also recognized the following principles needed for an NOF framework: Education and practice partnerships are crucial to develop an effective model; education and practice leaders must develop a collaborative model for achieving the minimum of a baccalaureate degree in nursing; create a more effective educational system to meet current and future health care needs; be proficient in a core set of competencies; and nurse educators in education and practice will use different teaching strategies to integrate NOF competencies into the curriculum (MDHE, 2010).

More information on the Nurse of the Future can be found at http://www.mass.edu/currentinit/NiNofCompetencies.asp.

THE ESSENTIALS OF BACCALAUREATE EDUCATION FOR PROFESSIONAL NURSING PRACTICE

The Essentials of Baccalaureate Education for Professional Nursing Practice (American Association of Colleges of Nursing [AACN], 2008a) is a set of central standards for baccalaureate-degree nursing education programs. As a framework for creating baccalaureate nursing programs, this document presents a comprehensive outline of expectations regarding basic knowledge, values, and professional behaviors of bachelor's-degree nursing graduates.

Essentials Standards I through IX describe in detail the outcomes expected of graduates of baccalaureate nursing programs. Achievement of these outcomes enables graduates to "practice within complex health care systems and assume the roles of provider of care; designer/manager/coordinator of care; and member of the profession" (AACN, 2008b).

The nine essentials are:

- Essential I: Liberal Education for Baccalaureate Generalist Nursing Practice
- Essential II: Basic Organizational and Systems Leadership for Quality Care and Patient Safety
- Essential III: Scholarship for Evidence-Based Practice
- Essential IV: Information Management and Application of Patient Care Technology
- Essential V: Healthcare Policy, Finance, and Regulatory Environments
- Essential VI: Interprofessional Communication and Collaboration for Improving Patient Health Outcomes
- Essential VII: Clinical Prevention and Population Health
- Essential VIII: Professionalism and Professional Values
- Essential IX: Baccalaureate Generalist Nursing Practice

The Essentials provide standards for preparing the baccalaureate-educated nurse to take on the various roles of caregiver, manager of care, and member of the profession. In addition, the document presents detailed standards for the educational requisites of liberal arts, role development, and basic knowledge "essential" for all baccalaureate nursing programs.

The Baccalaureate Essentials Tool Kit is a faculty resource for applying *The Essentials of Baccalaureate Education for Professional Nursing Practice* (AACN, 2008a). This document includes a review of the nine Baccalaureate Essentials followed by Integrative Learning Strategies, Opportunities for Program Enhancement, Web Links, AACN Presentations, and References. *The Essentials of Baccalaureate Education for Professional Nursing Practice* can be found at http://www.aacn.nche.edu/education-resources; www.aacn.nche.edu/publications/baccalaureate-toolkit.

AMERICAN ASSOCIATION OF COLLEGES OF NURSING (AACN)

The AACN advocates for baccalaureate and graduate nursing education. The AACN (2008b) has developed documents defining competency expectations for graduates of baccalaureate, master's, and doctor of nursing practice (DNP) programs. The AACN has also published quality indicators for research-focused doctoral programs, a white paper on the Clinical Nurse Leader (CNL), and guidelines defining essential clinical resources for nursing education, research, and faculty practice.

In its work on advancing public policy for nursing education, research, and practice, the AACN has acquired federal support for nursing education and research, guaranteeing continuing financial assistance for nursing students. An extension of the AACN, the Commission on Collegiate Nursing Education (CCNE) ensures the quality and integrity of baccalaureate and graduate education programs that are preparing effective nurses. As a national accreditation agency, the CCNE serves the public interest by assessing and identifying programs that engage in effective educational practices.

Annually, the AACN surveys all baccalaureate and graduate nursing programs, presenting data on student enrollments and graduations, faculty salaries, budgets, and institutional resources. Additionally, the AACN pursues grant funding to promote projects of special interest to nurse educators employed in baccalaureate education. The organization's current projects include incorporation of the CNL role into the health care delivery system, advocating for the adoption of nurse residency programs, and facilitating the transition to the DNP.

Additional information about the AACN can be found at www.aacn .nche.edu.

NURSING SHORTAGE

The United States Bureau of Labor Statistics (2012) reported that job growth in health care was responsible for one out of every five new jobs. Hospitals, long-term care facilities, and other ambulatory care settings added 49,000 new jobs in February 2012, up from 43,300 new jobs created in January.

As the largest segment of the health care workforce, RNs will likely be recruited to fill many of these new positions. In 2000, it was estimated that there were 110,000 open nursing positions, with demand exceeding supply by 6%. By 2025, the shortage of RNs is projected to reach an estimated 260,000, twice as high as any U.S. nursing shortage since the 1960s (Buerhaus, Auerbach, & Staiger, 2009).

The current shortage of nurses in the United states is linked with population growth, a shrinking pipeline of nursing students, a decline in RN earnings when compared with other careers, an aging labor force, as well as a growing, aging population in need of health care services (AACN, 2012).

Buerhaus and colleagues (2009) found that more than 75% of RNs believe the nursing shortage presents a major problem for the quality of their work life, the quality of client care, and the amount of time nurses can spend with clients. Surveyed nurses predict that shortages will increase stress on nurses, lead to a reduction in the quality of client care (93%), and inevitably cause nurses to leave the profession (93%).

Nursing shortages have been associated with medical errors (Aiken, Clarke, Sloane, Lake, & Cheney, 2008). Conversely, clients relate positive experiences in settings staffed by nurses who report job satisfaction. This is defined by a supportive working environment; positive nurse–physician relationships; administrative and collegial collaboration; and appropriate, safe nurse–client ratios. Where standards are ignored, with a practice environment of nurse turnover and understaffing, client mortality rates are higher. In a 2011 study, Blegen and other investigators found that higher nurse staffing levels were associated with fewer deaths, lower failure-to-rescue incidents, lower rates of infection, and shorter hospital stays (Blegen, Goode, Spetz, Vaughn, & Park, 2011).

Addressing the nursing shortage requires increased efforts toward recruitment and retention of nurses. According to the AACN's 2011 to 2012 report, *Enrollment and Graduations in Baccalaureate and Graduate Programs in Nursing*, U.S. nursing schools turned away 75,587 qualified applicants from baccalaureate and graduate nursing programs in 2011. Reasons included budget restraints, along with insufficient numbers of faculty, clinical sites, classroom space, and clinical preceptors (AACN, 2012). Although the AACN reported a 5.1% enrollment increase in entry-level baccalaureate programs in nursing in 2011, these statistics are a far cry from the numbers required to meet the anticipated need for nurses.

Strategies for confronting the nursing shortage include supplying academia with increased numbers of faculty and funding, enhancing student financial aid, and supporting the nontraditional student's pursuit of a career in nursing. Additional priorities include improving workplace conditions and providing the educational and professional development needed for career advancement, role satisfaction, and, ultimately, job retention.

In the IOM/RWJF report, *The Future of Nursing* (2010), the authors recommend encouraging nurses to practice to the fullest extent of their education and training, improving educational programs for nurses at every level to provide progression toward advanced degrees, and supporting nurses' memberships in health care reform debates. The report noted that nurses are often excluded from such decision-making boards. Including their input is viewed as invaluable to achieve improved morale and satisfaction among nurses.

ADVANCED PRACTICE

Advanced practice nursing has flourished in response to managed care. From changes in health care financing, society, and demographic populations, new advanced practice roles have developed and former roles have been transformed.

An advanced practice registered nurse (APRN) is a nurse with postgraduate education in nursing. APRNs have advanced didactic and clinical education, knowledge, skills, and scope of practice in nursing. APRN defines a level of nursing practice that utilizes extended and expanded skills, experience, and knowledge in assessment, planning, implementation, diagnosis, and evaluation of the care required. Nurses practicing at this level are educationally prepared at the postgraduate level and may work in either a specialist or generalist capacity (AACN, 2006).

APRNs demonstrate integration of theory, practice, and clinical experience. The educational experience is designed to empower the APRN to use multiple approaches to decision making; manage the care of individuals and groups; engage in collaborative practices with the client to achieve best outcomes; provide a supportive environment for colleagues; manage the utilization of staff and physical resources; engage in ethically justifiable nursing practice; protect the rights of individuals and groups; engage in activities to improve nursing practice; develop therapeutic and caring relationships; fulfill the conduct requirements of the profession; act to enhance the professional development of self; and function in accordance with legislation and common law affecting nursing practice (AACN, 2006).

APRN education encompasses 4 areas of specialization: nurse anesthetists, nurse midwives, clinical nurse specialists, and nurse practitioners. Each nurse specialty may have subspecialties or concentrations in a specific field or client population in health care. While education, accreditation, and certification are necessary elements of preparation for APRN practice, roles are regulated by legislation and specific professional regulation. This sustains prescribing and referral, insurance reimbursement, and admitting privileges to health care facilities. Licensing boards are governed by state regulations and statutes, and are the final authorities regarding those recognized to practice within a given state.

APRNs are required to attain at least a master's degree, generally a Master of Science in Nursing in their field of concentration. In 2004, the AACN and the National Council of State Boards of Nursing (NCSBN) recommended that APRNs move the entry-level degree to the doctorate level by 2015. All APRN training programs are required to transfer their master's degree to a DNP degree by the year 2015.

CHAPTER 3 REFLECTIVE QUESTIONS

1. What is the current view of quality and safety in both nursing practice and nursing education? Do you see it applied in your daily practice? If yes, how? If no, how would you, as a future baccalaureate-prepared nurse and leader, incorporate these competencies into health care organizations?

2. Compare Quality and Safety Education for Nurses (QSEN) and Nurse of the Future (NOF) initiatives. How are they alike/different? Why do you think they have been created and what is their significance to the profession?

3. How are the ANA standards incorporated into your nursing practice? Give examples.

4. After reading the section on the Institute of Medicine (IOM) report, what changes can you envision on your part to improve the workplace?

5. Refer to the documents published by the American Association of Colleges of Nursing (AACN), *The Baccalaureate Essentials Tool Kit* and *The Essentials of Baccalaureate Education for Professional Nursing Practice*. As a future baccalaureate-prepared nurse, why do you think it is important to understand and familiarize yourself with these documents and with professional nursing organizations such as the AACN and the Commission on Collegiate Nursing Education (CCNE)?

PART II

Core Competencies for the Baccalaureate-Prepared Nurse

Critical Thinking, the Nursing Process, and Evidence-Based Practice

OBJECTIVES

1. Explain why critical thinking skills are essential to nursing practice.
2. Identify the purposes of the nursing process.
3. Review the steps of the nursing process.
4. Describe the correlation of critical thinking, the nursing process, and evidence-based practice in nursing practice.
5. Compare care plan and concept map activities.
6. Recognize the influence of critical thinking/nursing process in regard to test-taking strategies.

KEY TERMS

Assessment

Clinical reasoning

Concept mapping

Critical thinking

Defining characteristics

Evaluation

Evidence-based nursing practice

Implementation

Item

Nursing care plan

Nursing diagnosis

Nursing process

PES statement

Planning

Stem

The Joint Commission (TJC)

STANDARDS

Evidence-Based Practice (EBP)		
Definition: Integrate best current evidence with clinical expertise and patient/family preferences and values for delivery of optimal health care.		
Knowledge	**Skills**	**Attitudes**
Demonstrate knowledge of basic scientific methods and processes. Describe EBP to include the components of research evidence, clinical expertise, and patient/family values	Participate effectively in appropriate data collection and other research activities. Adhere to institutional review board (IRB) guidelines Base individualized care plan on patient values, clinical expertise, and evidence	Appreciate strengths and weaknesses of scientific bases for practice. Value the need for ethical conduct of research and quality improvement Value the concept of EBP as integral to determining best clinical practice
Differentiate clinical opinion from research and evidence summaries. Describe reliable sources for locating evidence reports and clinical practice guidelines	Read original research and evidence reports related to area of practice. Locate evidence reports related to clinical practice topics and guidelines	Appreciate the importance of regularly reading relevant professional journals
Explain the role of evidence in determining best clinical practice. Describe how the strength and relevance of available evidence influence the choice of interventions in provision of patient-centered care	Participate in structuring the work environment to facilitate integration of new evidence into standards of practice. Question rationale for routine approaches to care that result in less-than-desired outcomes or adverse events	Value the need for continuous improvement in clinical practice based on new knowledge
Discriminate between valid and invalid reasons for modifying evidence-based clinical practice based on clinical expertise or patient/family preferences	Consult with clinical experts before deciding to deviate from evidence-based protocols	Acknowledge own limitations in knowledge and clinical expertise before determining when to deviate from evidence-based best practices

The most important practical lesson that can be given to nurses is to teach them what to observe—how to observe—what symptoms indicate improvement—what the reverse—which are of importance—which are of none—which are evidence of neglect—and of what kind of neglect. All this is what ought to make part, and an essential part, of the training of every nurse.

Florence Nightingale

I cannot teach anybody anything, I can only make them think.

Socrates, Greek philosopher

CRITICAL THINKING SKILLS

I am fortunate to have worked as an LPN...that's where I gained most of my critical thinking skills regarding crisis situations such as codes. I worked in a state veteran's hospital, and there were at least two codes per shift. If you were assigned to the code team that shift, it was your responsibility to attend each code. Codes are amazing...you truly see the team effort. Time simply vanishes, and it seems that you blink, and it's an hour later. You can read about codes, but it's when you actually experience them [that] they begin to make sense. I don't think anybody feels totally confident during every code. But like anything else, experience brings proficiency. Those experiences as an LPN have truly contributed to a wealth of knowledge in my career. Learning never ends.

Nursing student

This chapter explores the application of critical thinking, nursing process, and current evidence as a foundation for informed, safe, and professional nursing practice. The American Nurses Association (ANA, 2005) Standards provide the framework necessary for critical thinking in the application of the nursing process. The nursing process is a tool that fosters the nurse's proficiency in critical thinking.

Critical thinking is vital to evidence-based nursing practice. It supports nursing care and contributes to positive client outcomes across a variety of settings and geographic locations. The nature of evidence-based practice, its relevance to nursing, and the skills needed to support it are essential components of baccalaureate nursing education, all of which lead to the development of independent, self-directed learners, and, ultimately, professional nurses.

EVIDENCE-BASED NURSING PRACTICE

Evidence-based nursing is the practice of making clinical decisions based on the best available current research evidence, clinical expertise, and the needs and preferences of the client (Melnyk, Fineout-Overholt, Stillwell, & Williamson, 2009). It involves using sound, pertinent information for decision making in health care. This practice examines research findings, quality improvement data, and expert opinion. Moreover, it challenges nurses to look at the "why" behind present systems, existing methods, and processes in the search for improvement. Key steps in the evidence-based practice process involve:

1. Formulating a clinical question
2. Gathering the best evidence to answer the clinical question
3. Critically appraising the best evidence
4. Integrating the evidence with the provider's expertise, assessment of the client's condition, values and preferences, and available health care resources in order to make a clinical decision
5. Evaluating the practice change as a result of applying the evidence

While all of the steps are essential, the fifth is often the one most neglected (Melnyk, Fineout-Overholt, Stillwell, & Williamson, 2009). It is not uncommon for practitioners to implement a practice change based on evidence but fail to evaluate the effectiveness of the change. Evaluation of the practice change is vital in order to disseminate effectiveness of a treatment or clinical decision change to other health care professionals.

Client care must be based on evidence for optimal outcomes. Equally as important as utilizing evidence as the foundation of quality patient care is the conduct of research to fill the gaps in existing nursing literature. While nurses can be educated about implementing evidence-based practice at the bedside, continual encouragement is necessary from nursing administration (Melnyk, Fineout-Overholt, Gallagher-Ford, & Stillwell, 2011). This support is vital in achieving an evidence-based practice culture in the nursing profession.

THE NURSING PROCESS AND CARE PLANNING

A care plan documents the nursing process, defines an organized problem-solving approach to the client's individual needs, and prioritizes nursing problems (Gordon, 2010). The nursing process is a critical thinking, problem-solving method based on the scientific method used by the various science disciplines in proving or disproving theories. Beginning nursing students use the "long form" by creating nursing care plans for assigned clients in the clinical setting.

By taking the time to pull apart the process, students begin to understand its components. With continued exposure to the process, students come to realize that this organized approach is applicable to every aspect of the nursing profession. With experience in practice, nurses carry the "short form" of the nursing care plan in their heads.

The nurse identifies the client's needs **(problem; P)** by first completing a thorough assessment. From this assessment, the nurse begins to identify problems/nursing diagnoses, which are related to **(etiology; E)** dysfunction in a particular area. The client's abnormal data identified during the assessment provides the basis for **signs and symptoms (S**), labeled by the North American Nursing Diagnosis Association (NANDA) as **defining characteristics**. Nurses must be able to defend their choice of a nursing diagnosis with a comprehensive, sound assessment.

Simply stated, the nursing care plan commits the critical thinking process to paper (Table 4.1). Regardless of format (concept mapping, standardized, handwritten, or computer-generated), the nursing care plan is part of the client's legal record. The nurse is responsible for addressing and documenting in the client's record those problems identified as nursing diagnoses, the human response to the client's medical diagnosis (Gordon, 2010).

According to guidelines from The Joint Commission (TJC), the care planning process is the structural framework for coordinating communication that will result in safe and effective care. *The Essentials of Baccalaureate Education for Professional Nursing Practice*, drafted by the accrediting body the American Association of Colleges of Nursing (AACN, 2008a), lists several core competencies that directly relate to the nurse's care planning process, including the ability to ". . . diagnose, plan, deliver, and evaluate quality care" (p. 11), "use appropriate technologies in the process of assessing and monitoring patients" (p. 14), "apply health care technologies to maximize optimal outcomes for patients" (p. 16), and "develop a comprehensive plan of care . . ." (p. 16).

Each nursing diagnosis has its own set of symptoms. They are listed in the NANDA taxonomy sections of texts, which can be found in the reference section here. As students begin to learn the language of the nursing process, or ADPIE (assessment, diagnosis, planning, implementation, and evaluation), their challenge is to write the problem statement in its appropriate format: problem, etiology, signs and symptoms (PES).

The following information related to the nursing process takes the writer through each step when creating a written care plan:

1. **Assessment**: In this phase the nurse interviews the client, collects data from the medical record, completes a physical assessment, and reviews current literature related to the client's medical diagnosis, as well as signs, symptoms, and pathophysiology.

2. **Determination of the patient's problem(s)/nursing diagnosis**: Here the nurse reviews the assessment findings to identify any dysfunction, translating the problem to a NANDA-approved nursing diagnosis. From here the nurse formulates the diagnosis using the aforementioned PES format. However, "Risk for" nursing diagnostic statements contain only "P" and "E," as the behavior ("S") has not been exhibited at this point.

3. **Planning**: In this phase, the nurse writes realistic, prioritized, and measurable long- and short-term goals/outcomes. Note that in the planning stage, both the nurse and the client work **together** to achieve these goals. These goals are client-based—"The client will (verbalize, demonstrate . . .)"—using action verbs. Interventions to assist in meeting these goals are spelled out here.

4. **Implementation**: This is the action or "doing" phase, in which the actual plan is carried out in order to meet the goals for the client.

5. **Evaluation**: In determining if the goals/outcomes have been met, the nurse asks the following questions: Have the goals been totally met, partially met, or not met? How can the nurse modify the plan to achieve the goals?

TABLE 4.1 Nursing Care Plan Example With Instructor Feedback

Gordon Functional Health Pattern	Assessments (Text resource: Ackley & Ladwig, 2011)	Did you identify any problems from the assessment in any of the patterns below? If so, formulate an appropriate nursing diagnosis, using the "PES" format (Problem, Etiology, Signs and Symptoms.) Note: "Risk for" statements: "P" & "E" only.
		Problem/Nursing Diagnosis Identified? No problems noted in this pattern.
1. Health Perception/ Health Maintenance	Allergies/ how allergies manifest themselves in client: 1. No allergies 2. During the pregnancy how much caffeine (coffee, tea, soda) is consumed daily: 2 cups of coffee/day; no soda	
	Smoke: No	
	If so, how many per day?	
	Anyone in the home smoke? No	
	How much alcohol typically consumed: None	
	Current or past use/abuse of other substances: None	
	Current medications: Name, dose, and reason for taking: Prenatal vitamins, 1 tab daily Ibuprofen (Motrin) 600 mg PO q 6 hr PRN for pain 3–4 Docusate Sodium (Colace) 100 mg PO BID PRN for constipation Dibucain Ointment PRN for perineal pain > 3 Tucks Pad PRN for perineal pain > 3	
	Pre-existing medical conditions: None	

(continued)

TABLE 4.1 Nursing Care Plan Example With Instructor Feedback (*continued*)

	Problem/Nursing Diagnosis Identified?
Client's age: 29	
Marital status: married	
Ethnicity: Caucasian/American Indian	
Date began prenatal care: August 2, 2012	
Attended all scheduled visits? Yes	
If not, why?	
Childbirth classes: Yes	
Reaction to pregnancy (client): Excited	
Reaction to pregnancy (SO): Nervous	
Reaction to pregnancy (children): N/A	
Exposure to teratogens during pregnancy? No	
Risk factors for this pregnancy: Family history of diabetes, hypertension, cleft palate, bipolar disorder	
Complications of previous pregnancies: None	
Prenatal labs	
Blood type (ABO): B	
Rh type: Positive	
Results of Glucola: 101	
Follow-up needed? No	
VDRL: Nonreactive	
Gonorrhea culture: Negative	
HIV: Negative	
Rubella titer: Non-immune	

(*continued*)

TABLE 4.1 Nursing Care Plan Example With Instructor Feedback *(continued)*

Hepatitis B screen:	Negative
GBS status:	Negative
If GBS status positive or unknown: Treated?	
With number of treatments: No treatment needed	
History of protein or glucose in prenatal urine: Negative	
H&H – prenatal: 14.6% and 39% H&H day after delivery:	

		Problem/Nursing Diagnosis Identified?
2. Nutrition/Metabolic	VS. T: 36.4 P: 79 R: 15 B/P: 125/78	**SIGNIFICANT**
	Oxygen saturation: 98%	
	Lung sounds: Clear	
	Ht: 64 inches	
	Pregnancy weight gain: 48 lbs	
	Pre-pregnancy weight: 210 lbs	
	BMI: 43	
	Spacings between pregnancies: No previous	
	pregnancy	
	Lacerations or episiotomy? 2nd degree laceration	
	Perineal swelling/bruising: Perineal swelling	
	Surgical incision? (dressing): None	
	Postpartum IV fluids? No (What is infusing, rate):	
	Saline lock? No	
	Does client have annual dental exams/cleanings? Yes	
	Teeth even, no visible decay	

(continued)

TABLE 4.1 Nursing Care Plan Example With Instructor Feedback (*continued*)

	Problem/Nursing Diagnosis Identified?
Typical eating schedule? No restrictions to diet. Where are meals usually eaten? At home; dinner out once a week.	
Example of a meal in a typical day:	
Breakfast: Cereal and fruit	
Lunch: Sandwich, soup, water	
Dinner: Meat, vegetable, rice	
Fluids: Water and coffee	
Client's perception of diet: States she has "a good appetite."	
Client consumed 100% of breakfast	
Diet/nutrition education	
Does client request information? No	
Does client need education? (explain) Nutrition while breastfeeding	
Outcomes to education provided: Client understood that there were no contraindications for diet	
Appetite since delivery? Ate 100% of breakfast	
Assessment of breasts	**Ineffective breastfeeding related to (R/T) flat nipples as evidenced by (AEB) pt. using breast shield and infant difficulty maintaining latch.**
If bottlefeeding – aware of care of breasts? Teaching provided?	**Readiness for enhanced learning R/T breastfeeding AEB mother's request for assistance with breastfeeding.**
If breastfeeding:	
Mother's ability to position infant at breast:	
Adequate; used position that was most comfortable (football), required a nipple shield for flat nipples	
Maternal effort/desire to maintain lactation: Adequate	

(continued)

TABLE 4.1 Nursing Care Plan Example With Instructor Feedback *(continued)*

		Problem/Nursing Diagnosis:
	(requested assistance with feeding) Newborn's ability to latch properly: Ineffective; inability to maintain latch Regular and sustained suckling/swallowing at breast: Ineffective; inability to maintain latch Does the infant appear content after nursing? (describe behavior): Did not observe successful feed	
3. Elimination	Bowel pattern prior to pregnancy: Last BM: Before labor Bowel sounds present? Yes Passing flatus: Yes Constipation/diarrhea during pregnancy Hemorrhoids: No History UTIs: No Indwelling Foley catheter: No First void 4/1 2358 hr	**SIGNIFICANT**

(continued)

TABLE 4.1 Nursing Care Plan Example With Instructor Feedback (*continued*)

4. Activity Exercise	Problem/Nursing Diagnosis Identified?
Is client reporting decreased energy, feeling drowsy or tired? Patient reported that she was tired, and didn't sleep the night previously	**Fatigue R/T noise AEB patient reports little sleep due to infant crying.**
What, if any, medical conditions affect client's ability to exercise? None	
Prior to pregnancy did client engage in regular exercise (30 minutes or more of physical activity/exercise at least 2–3 days a week)? Yes	
If yes, what type of activity? Walking	
Was exercise pattern modified during pregnancy? No	
Motivation to exercise? Anxious to return to exercise	
Do work/family demands impact ability to engage in exercise or recreational activities? No	
Resources to engage in physical activities? Yes	
How is leisure time spent? With family and friends	

(continued)

TABLE 4.1 Nursing Care Plan Example With Instructor Feedback (*continued*)

		Problem/Nursing Diagnosis Identified?
5. Cognitive/Perceptual	Language spoken: English Does the client report any pain or discomfort? No pain reported. Patient reports feeling "discomfort but no pain." Pain scale (0–10): 0 Guarding behaviors: No Grimacing: No Muscle tension: None Is client managing pain effectively? Patient using ice to perineal area from laceration during labor. Patient reports this measure as effective. **Pharmacological management:** Patient-controlled analgesia (PCA) (Medication/settings): No Oral medications for pain: Name, dose, effectiveness (0–10 scale) Ibuprofen (Motrin) 600 mg PO q 6 hr for pain PRN Nonpharmacological interventions: Ice to perineum applied first 24 hrs **Educational needs:** What does the client know about newborn care? Client and father of baby (FOB) report taking the childbirth education classes and staff has provided education per teaching sheet. Basic knowledge about nutrition, breastfeeding, infant care What information does the client request (teaching sheet or your assessment)?	**PAIN R/T vaginal birth. AEB patient reports discomfort, uses an ice pack to relieve discomfort in perineum.**

(continued)

TABLE 4.1 Nursing Care Plan Example With Instructor Feedback (*continued*)

	Problem/Nursing Diagnosis Identified?
Client requests information about weaning her baby from a nipple shield. Father requests information about when the best time is to breastfeed their baby. No breastfeeding class attended.	**Readiness for enhanced knowledge R/T postpartum newborn and breastfeeding education AEB parental statements regarding breastfeeding**
What information did you provide your client related to newborn care (teaching sheet or your assessment)? Return of menses, exercise/rest, breast care/ engorgement, nutrition, family planning, sexual relations, jaundice/bilirubin, SIDS, temp. axillary, infant cues, feeding positions, frequency/duration, latch on/off, frequency/ amounts during feeds.	
What information did you provide your client related to postpartum self-care (teaching sheet or your assessment)? Perineum care, ambulation	
Does the client verbalize an understanding of what was taught? Yes	
Are there any barriers to teaching? FATIGUE	

(*continued*)

TABLE 4.1 Nursing Care Plan Example With Instructor Feedback (*continued*)

		Problem/Nursing Diagnosis Identified?
6. Sleep/Rest	Does the client report feeling fatigue or exhibit signs of fatigue (yawning, rubbing eyes, signs of irritability)? Patient seems fatigued from inability to sleep the night of delivery Did the client sleep last night? Limited sleep If not, why? Crying baby Difficulty with sleep prior to pregnancy? No Usual sleep pattern? Unknown Naps? Yes	**Fatigue R/T noise AEB patient reports little sleep due to infant crying.**
7. Coping/Stress Tolerance	Does client report increase of life stress or problems? No Does she believe the new stressors are manageable? Unknown Does the client report feeling anxious or depressed? Anxious about being ineffective at breastfeeding How does the client usually manage stress, anxiety, or depression (coping mechanisms)? Talking with her family, friends, and husband Are her usual coping mechanisms effective now? (If not, explain): Yes Does the client request additional support to manage additional stressors? No If so, what services are offered to client? Does client have a support system? Yes If so, identify members of support system: Husband, family, and friends	**ANXIETY R/T threat to role function AEB patient verbalized that she is anxious about being ineffective at breastfeeding.**

(*continued*)

TABLE 4.1 Nursing Care Plan Example With Instructor Feedback (*continued*)

	Problem/Nursing Diagnosis Identified?
Is client's primary support person providing sufficient support to manage the additional stressors? Husband; yes What bonding stages are noted with infant? Taking in/ taking hold Who is bonding with infant? Mother and father Help at home with infant/siblings? Yes Symptoms of or history of postpartum blues or depression: No previous pregnancies	
8. Self-Perception/ Self-Concept	
Does the client report feeling anxious about her role (first-time mother, the additional responsibility of another child, being a single parent): Anxious about breastfeeding If so, how is she managing the anxiety? Talking with staff and husband about ways to effectively feed. Attempting different breastfeeding positions and using nipple shield. What services will be offered to client? Information sheet provided to client on breastfeeding support group offered and lactation consultant during hospital stay Does the client verbalize concerns about the changes to her body? No How is she coping with the changes? N/A (not applicable) Does client make eye contact when speaking? Yes Assessment of patient's self-perception/self-concept: Patient presents as excited about her new role as a mother; however, states she is very tired from not being able to sleep that night	

(continued)

TABLE 4.1 Nursing Care Plan Example With Instructor Feedback (*continued*)

		Problem/Nursing Diagnosis Identified?
9. Role/Relationship	Does client appear to accept the change in her role responsibilities? Yes	
	If not, explain:	
	Is the mother physically, emotionally, and financially prepared to care for her newborn/family members? Yes	
	If not, explain:	
	Who does the client live with? (list all members of household): Husband and newborn	
	FOB involved: Yes	
	Interaction of parenting couple: Kind and caring toward each other and infant	
	Interaction of family members: Kind, caring, and positive support	
	Adequate resources to provide required care? Yes	
	Mother's occupation: Project Manager	
	Plan to return to work? Yes—has designated breastfeeding rooms in workplace. When? 3 months	
	Child care arranged? Not yet	
	Children: 0 Ages:	
	Do they live at home?	
	Are siblings prepared for the baby? No siblings; firstborn	
	Need of support services? None. WIC: VNA:	
	OTHER:	

(continued)

TABLE 4.1 Nursing Care Plan Example With Instructor Feedback (*continued*)

		Problem/Nursing Diagnosis Identified?
10. Sexuality/ Reproductive	Last menstrual period (LMP): Unsure	
	Did the client require induction or augmentation of labor? No	
	Time of spontaneous repture of membranes (SROM): 3/31 6 a.m.	
	Description of amniotic fluid: Clear	
	Time and type of delivery: Spontaneous vaginal delivery at 0111 4/1	
	Presentation: Vertex	
	Complications? None	
	Is client currently involved in an intimate relationship? Yes	
	If so, what are plans for birth control? IUD	
	Does the client verbalize any problems in sexual relationships? No	
	Fundus (height/firmness): Firm, 1 cm below umbilicus	
	Lochia (type/amount): Small, rubra	
11. Values/ Beliefs	Client's religious affiliation: Protestant	**Problem/Nursing Diagnosis Identified?**
	Does client currently practice her religion? Nonaffiliated	
	What is perceived as important in life? Family	
	Are there any perceived conflicts in values or beliefs that are health-related? None	

(*continued*)

TABLE 4.1 Nursing Care Plan Example With Instructor Feedback (*continued*)

Date and Time of Delivery: 4/1/2013, 0111; Type of Delivery: vaginal; Infant: female X̲ male

NURSING CARE PLAN: You must defend your choice of nursing diagnosis/diagnoses with a thorough assessment (above) that identifies and documents those problem areas noted in a particular health care pattern.

NURSING DIAGNOSIS	INTERVENTIONS	RATIONALE FOR EACH INTERVENTION	EXPECTED GOAL/OUTCOME	EVALUATION
Readiness for enhanced knowledge R/T postpartum newborn and breastfeeding education AEB parental statements regarding breastfeeding (Ackley & Ladwig, 2011, p. 521)	(cite each intervention with author, year, page number/s) 1. ASSESS KNOWLEDGE LEVEL	(cite each rationale with author, year, page number/s) 1.	Client expresses knowledge on where to obtain information and support for breastfeeding by discharge	Client can locate information for breastfeeding support
	2. ASSESS READINESS TO LEARN	2.	Client expresses understanding of methods to facilitate breastfeeding by discharge	Client can demonstrate methods to facilitate breastfeeding
	3. ASSESS PAIN LEVEL	3.		Client can verbalize rationale for infant care
	4. OBSERVE AN ENTIRE BREASTFEEDING SESSION	4.	Client expresses understanding of rationale for infant care by discharge	Client verbalizes increased understanding of breastfeeding and infant care
	5. Include clients as members of health care team in goal setting when providing education (CITATION) HOW DOES THIS R/T YOUR CLIENT?	5. Involving clients is relevant, meaningful to them, and important component of supporting client participation (CITATION)		

(continued)

TABLE 4.1 Nursing Care Plan Example With Instructor Feedback (*continued*)

6. Support client priorities, preferences, and choice (CITATION) HOW DOES THIS R/T YOUR CLIENT? SPECIFY	6. Supporting client priorities, preferences, and choices facilitates education with client cooperation and promotes patient autonomy (CITATION)
7. Seek teachable moments to encourage health promotion (CITATION) HOW DOES THIS R/T YOUR CLIENT?	7. Use teachable moments to offer information on health promotion and prevention behaviors (CITATION)
8. Individualize health education interventions WHAT DO YOU MEAN BY THIS? ELABORATE HERE. HOW DOES THIS RELATE SPECIFICALLY TO YOUR CLIENT? (CITATION)	8. Interventions tailored to the learning needs of the client positively affect lifestyle changes (CITATION)
9. Encourage group and peer support as appropriate to enhance learning (Ackley & Ladwig, 2011, p. 522)	9. Peer support instrumental in enhancing client knowledge, skills, confidence (Ackley & Ladwig, 2011, p. 522)
10. Reinforce learning through educational follow-up (Ackley & Ladwig, 2011, p. 523) WHAT DOES THIS MEAN AS IT R/T YOUR CLIENT?	10. Longer periods of participation over time; consistent structured educational programs have resulted in symptom management and risk reduction (Ackley & Ladwig, 2011, p. 523)

REFLECTION

1. **Describe three interactions with staff/client/peers that helped you to feel more independent/confident in your nursing practice.**

   During the clinical day, three interactions that helped me feel more independent and confident in my nursing practice were providing teaching to the patient and her husband, reporting to the nurse, and how I was able to prioritize care for the patient. While I was teaching the patient and her husband, I surprised myself because I knew what I was talking about, and was providing solid, reliable information. When reporting to the nurse, I was able to prioritize what was most important and relevant to the care of my patient. This told me I understand what is truly important in patient care, and what is important for the nurse to know about a patient. In addition, I was able to make a list of what I needed to do for the patient; prioritized what had to be done first, second, and third; and completed the most important aspects of patient care during the day (vital signs, physical assessment).

2. **Identify three areas of your performance during this clinical day that you felt were strong.**

   Three areas during the clinical day that I felt were strong were my teaching abilities, vital signs and adult assessment, and my ability to speak with and interact with my patient. I have no problem providing teaching to people; I find myself doing it with friends, coworkers, and customers at work, and, since I work in the service industry, I have no issues interacting with a variety of people of various racial and ethnic groups who speak a variety of languages and practice various customs. In addition, I have had a lot of experience assessing adults, and I am confident in my ability to assess the condition of an adult.

3. **Identify three areas of your performance during this clinical day that you feel need improvement.**

   Three areas of my performance during the clinical day that I would like to improve upon are documentation and charting, infant assessment, and infant care (diaper change, vital signs). Additional experience charting is key to developing expertise, and I have not assessed infants or performed infant care enough to feel comfortable with it. WILL GET YOU THIS "PRACTICE" TO HELP YOU COMPLETE THIS OBJECTIVE AND FEEL MORE COMFORTABLE AND SELF-CONFIDENT IN THIS AREA.

CONCEPT MAPPING

More than ever, the expansion in current knowledge and technology surrounding health and health care requires the involvement of intelligent, creative, and innovative individuals. A significant responsibility for nurse educators is to empower graduates with critical thinking and problem-solving skills. If the ultimate goal of professional nursing is providing quality client care, nursing educators must use creative, innovative teaching methods that meet these needs (Taylor & Wros, 2007).

Concept mapping is an active teaching method that assists students in the acquisition of these competencies. A visual representation of relationships among concepts, this teaching approach is based on Ausubel's (2000) view that learning occurs when the individual is able to organize and relate the concepts and new information of cognitive mental structures. It is a concrete way to present how an individual mapper visualizes a particular topic. Concepts are characterized by single words enclosed in a box and connected to other concept boxes by arrows. A word or phrase defines the relationship between the connected concepts. Major concept boxes have lines to and from several other concept boxes, generating a network.

When constructing a concept map, the individual should first identify facts, terms, and ideas associated with the topic. List the items and print them on "sticky" notes, one per note. Spread out the concepts as notes on a flat surface for easy reading and to create related groups. Identify terms that represent higher categories and add them. Some concepts will fall into multiple groupings.

Arrange and rearrange in an order that best represents the understanding of the interrelationships and connections among groupings. Use a consistent hierarchy in which the most important concepts are in the center or at the top. Think in terms of connecting the items in a simple sentence that shows the relationship between them. Use lines with arrows to connect and show the relationship between connected items. Write a word or short phrase by each arrow to specify the relationship. Many arrows can originate or terminate on particularly important concepts.

In reviewing the completed concept map, Schuster (2008) recommends mappers consider the following characteristics:

> **Accuracy and Thoroughness.** Are the concepts and relationships correct? Are important concepts missing? Are any misconceptions apparent?

FIGURE 4.1 Concept Map Example

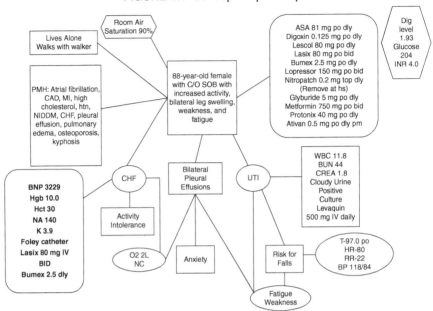

Organization. Was the concept map laid out in a way that higher-order relationships are apparent and easy to follow? Does it have a title?

Appearance. Was the assignment done with care, showing attention to details such as spelling and penmanship?

Creativity. Are there unusual elements that aid communication or stimulate interest without being distracting?

Concept maps are useful for summarizing information, consolidating information from different sources, thinking through complex problems, and presenting information (Figure 4.1).

CRITICAL THINKING, THE NURSING PROCESS, AND STRATEGIES FOR TEST TAKING

While test-taking skills are no replacement for good study habits, they can positively impact overall test performance. Memorizing facts is not enough. Most questions require a thorough understanding of the knowledge content measured by a test, as well as the use of higher, more complex thought processes.

Test scores are significantly influenced by reading aptitude. In answering a test item (the test question itself), begin by carefully reading the stem (that portion of the test item that poses the question). Consider what the test question is really asking. Look for key words in the stem, along with any information relevant to answering the question (Hogan, 2007).

After careful evaluation of the stem, consider the options (test answers listed). Look for an option that is similar to the answer you have chosen. Is this option the most suitable answer to the test question? Address the question as it is stated, without reading anything into it or making assumptions about it. Answer the question asked, not the one you would like to answer.

Certain key words in the stem, the options, or both should alert the test taker to the need for thoughtfulness in choosing your answer. Because few things are absolute without exception, avoid selecting answers that include words such as *always, never, all, every, only, must, no,* and *none.* Answers containing these key words are rarely correct because they place special limitations and qualifications on potentially correct answers (Hogan, 2007).

If the options in an item do not seem to make sense because more than one option is correct, reread the question: You may have missed one of the key words in the stem. Be aware when you see one of the key words in an option; it may limit the context in which such an option would be correct.

The well-written multiple-choice question is precisely stated, providing you with only the information needed to make the question or problem clear and specific. Careful reading of details in the stem can provide important clues to the correct option. Eliminate clearly incorrect, inappropriate, and unlikely answers to the question asked in the stem. By systematically eliminating distracters that are unlikely in the context of a given question, you increase the probability of selecting the correct answer. Eliminating obvious distracters also allows you more time to focus on the options that appear to be potentially sound answers to the question.

If uncertain about the correct answer to a question, it is better to make an educated guess than to not answer the question. The test taker can generally eliminate one or more of the distracters by using partial knowledge and the methods just listed. The elimination process increases your chances of selecting the correct option from those remaining. Elimination of two distracters on a four-option multiple-choice item increases your probability of selecting the correct answer from 25% to 50% (Hogan, 2007).

As you begin the exam, structure your testing time. Develop check points to stay on schedule. Answer easy questions first. If you are unsure of an answer, either give it your best shot and move on, or skip it and make a mark so you are sure to go back to it. Understand what the question is asking.

Test-Taking Tips

Anticipate the answer. Read the question thoroughly. Try and answer the question in your own words, then look at the options and see which alternative matches or is closest to your answer.

Read the stem and each alternative. Answer each alternative as true, false, or don't know. If you know the answer, choose it; don't look for tricks. Read the stem and the answer you've chosen together to see if they make sense. Ask yourself what the relationship is between the two choices. If the relationship is "set to subset," then one option is an *umbrella response*. If this is the case, pick the umbrella, because it includes the other answer. If the relationship isn't "set to subset," ask yourself which option is *most important* in that situation. What is the question really asking (Nugent & Vitale, 2011)?

Answer the condition in the stem. Is the question asking for a general or a specific answer? The phase "Which one of the following?" asks for a specific answer. "In general . . ." is asking for a broad overview or a general response.

Relate each option to the stem. Each option (a, b, c, d) should be grammatically correct and consistent. Your choice should "make sense" to you. Read the question and answer as a complete sentence.

Focus your reading. Read carefully. Don't be distracted by irrelevant or extraneous words or phrases. Rephrase the stem into your own words. Break the stem into critical elements and attack them separately. Ask: What is this really asking? How would you paraphrase this question to explain it to someone else?

Try not to overthink or "out-guess" the instructor. Read the question as it is actually written. If you know the answer, choose it. Don't think "It can't be that—that's too easy."

Do not change your answers. Go with your first hunch. Don't change your answer unless you have a *good reason* to do so.

Avoid "nursing student paranoia." If you see an unfamiliar term, don't assume it must be the correct answer. Students often think, "I don't know what that term means, so it must be the right answer." Learn all new terms to avoid this!

Remember the saying: "Practice makes perfect." As you are studying, do as many practice questions as possible. Use the nonproctored online exams from review books, sample tests, and NCLEX review books.

CHAPTER 4 REFLECTIVE QUESTIONS

1. Describe a "critical incident," an experience where you believe the intervention made a difference in a client outcome. Give a detailed description of what happened.

2. Discuss any experience you have had with nursing care plans and concept mapping. After reading further about these methods, which do you prefer and why? How does working with care plans/concept maps foster critical thinking in nursing?

3. Describe how critical thinking, the nursing process, and evidence-based practice "fit" together in caring for clients.

4. What have you observed related to evidence-based practice in your workplace? Why do you think it is important to have an evidence-based practice philosophy?

5. Which test-taking strategies work best for you? What might you add to your "repertoire" of strategies after reading this chapter?

CHAPTER 5

The Teaching and Learning Process in Nursing

OBJECTIVES

1. Examine the role of the nurse as teacher.
2. Discuss Knowles's assumptions regarding adult learners.
3. Analyze cognitive, affective, and psychomotor domains of learning.
4. Identify guidelines for effective teaching and learning.
5. Summarize Kolb's framework in the identification of learning styles.
6. Review the Visual–Auditory–Kinesthetic/Tactile Questionnaire.
7. Explain the concept of health literacy.
8. Critique a sample case study and teaching plan.

KEY TERMS

Accommodating	Learning theory
Affective	Learning styles
Assimilating	Psychomotor
Cognitive	Teach-back method
Converging	Teaching plan
Diverging	Visual Auditory, Read/Write,
Health literacy	Kinesthetic (VARK) Survey

STANDARDS

Quality Improvement (QI)		
Definition: Use data to monitor the outcomes of care processes and use improvement methods to design and test changes to continuously improve the quality and safety of health care systems.		
Knowledge	Skills	Attitudes
Describe strategies for learning about the outcomes of care in the setting in which one is engaged in clinical practice	Seek information about outcomes of care for populations served in care setting. Seek information about quality improvement projects in the care setting	Appreciate that continuous quality improvement is an essential part of the daily work of all health professionals
Recognize that nursing and other health professions students are parts of systems of care and care processes that affect outcomes for patients and families. Give examples of the tension between professional autonomy and system functioning	Use tools (such as flow charts, cause–effect diagrams) to make processes of care explicit. Participate in a root cause analysis of a sentinel event	Value own and others' contributions to outcomes of care in local care settings
Explain the importance of variation and measurement in assessing quality of care	Use quality measures to understand performance. Use tools (such as control charts and run charts) that are helpful for understanding variation. Identify gaps between local and best practice	Appreciate how unwanted variation affects care. Value measurement and its role in good patient care
Describe approaches for changing processes of care	Design a small test of change in daily work (using an experiential learning method such as Plan–Do–Study–Act). Practice aligning the aims, measures, and changes involved in improving care. Use measures to evaluate the effect of change	Value local change (in individual practice or team practice on a unit) and its role in creating joy in work. Appreciate the value of what individuals and teams can do to improve care

Teaching others has been a part of nursing for a long time (Nightingale, 1969). Client education is both an expectation and a legal obligation of the professional nurse (AACN, 2008a).

The purposes of client education are to maintain health, improve health, or slow declining health. Positive outcomes related to client education require effective communication skills in order to assess individual needs, attitudes, and preferences impacting health behaviors. In addition to communication and assessment skills, the nurse must have appropriate understanding of the information to be taught. If the knowledge base is lacking, the nurse risks client safety by delivering inadequate or inaccurate information (Falvo, 2011).

This chapter provides an introduction to the concepts related to the process of client education, describing the professional responsibilities that nurses, as lifelong learners, must possess not only for their own education, but for the teaching and learning needs of clients, families, colleagues, and the community. The topics of nurse as teacher, principles of adult learning, factors that interfere with teaching–learning, and effective methods of teaching are included.

TAKING THE TIME TO TEACH: A PERSONAL STORY

I was caring for a 75-year-old man recently admitted to our long-term care facility. He had diagnoses of chronic pain, mental illness, and kidney problems. I noted that both of his legs were very swollen. Any instructions I gave him to reduce the swelling, he challenged: I taught him to elevate (he doesn't because of chronic back pain), remain compliant with meds (he doesn't like taking his Lasix because he doesn't want to have to urinate "50 times a day") and to do his leg stretches ("Don't you remember I am in constant pain?"). I finally knelt down in front of him and said, "I want you to know I am very worried about you." He smiled at me and said, "Thank you so much for caring," and proceeded to tell me about what had happened that made him so angry, that no one really cared ("They've all given up on me."). I learned to stop judging the situation and see what was in front of me. I realized it didn't matter what I thought he should be doing; that to be an effective nurse and teacher I had to offer the care that he was able and willing to accept. I was able to show him that there were people in the health care field that genuinely wanted to help and really did care about his well-being. The intervention was quite simply sitting down and listening without one foot out the door. This is the type of health care I believe to be most beneficial for the individual.

Nursing student

Tell me and I forget. Teach me and I remember. Involve me and I learn.

Benjamin Franklin

TEACHING AND LEARNING IN NURSING

The purposes of client education are to maintain health, improve health, or slow the deterioration of health. Effective client education requires the nurse to have the ability to communicate effectively with clients to assess the individual needs, attitudes, and preferences of the client that can affect health behavior before any changes can be expected. Additionally, the nurse must understand how to teach clients and possess sufficient knowledge of the information that needs to be taught. Insufficient knowledge in these areas diminishes the nurse's credibility and ultimately the client's health (Falvo, 2011).

Teaching, "a planned activity designed to facilitate learning" (Rogers, 1969), and learning, "a change in behavior as a result of a learning experience" (Haggard, 1963), consist of providing accurate and consistent information, demonstrations, and guidance to clients, their families, or significant others regarding the client's health status and health. This is carried out for the purposes of increasing knowledge, assisting the client to reach an optimum level of health functioning and participation in self-care, and promoting the client's ability to make informed decisions. Additionally, it incorporates assessing the client's needs, abilities, and knowledge level; adapting teaching content and methods to the identified needs, abilities, and knowledge level of the client; evaluating effectiveness of teaching and counseling; and making referrals to appropriate resources.

As the "Father of Adult Education," Malcolm Knowles (1990) developed a body of work on learning theory and provided an important framework for teaching adults. Once understood, this information helps the nurse educator to approach client education from a perspective that will enable successful learning and lead to more effective client outcomes. Adult learning theory's premise is that there must be a change in the focus from the teacher to the learner. Teaching can be carried out in any number of ways, as long as learning is facilitated. The result is a teacher free to identify creative strategies to provide information to the patient without always being the direct medium for that information.

Knowles described five assumptions about adults as learners that have practical applications for teaching in the real world:

1. **Adults are self-directed.** Adult learners know what they want to know and expect to have some voice in the educational process. The nurse as teacher can create a climate of mutual respect by involving the learner in the process, encouraging feedback related to how the information is disseminated, and providing positive reinforcement.

2. **Adults have life experience that should be considered in their educational process.** By incorporating the learner's life skills and knowledge, the nurse as teacher establishes an environment of caring and respect. Creating such an atmosphere builds on the learner's previous knowledge and experience. Many clients admitted to the hospital for the first time bring with them valuable life experiences and accomplishments and are curious, somewhat wary, but invested in this unfamiliar setting.

3. **Adult learning is usually problem or role centered. Adults often engage in learning because of roles they currently assume in the family, work, or community; jobs they have or will have; or circumstances in which they find themselves.** If a nurse employs active listening skills, the client perceives the nurse's active listening as individualized caring. The client is viewed as a person, one outside the sick role. Additionally, by paying careful attention to those areas of the client's life considered by the client to be valued, the teacher (nurse) can effect a positive outcome related to the client's willingness to learn.

4. **Adults tend to be internally motivated. They rarely learn just because someone else, even a physician or a nurse, tells them it's important for them to do so.** It is critical for nurse–teachers to work diligently to enable understanding of the information taught for the well-being of both client and family. It may be necessary to involve family members to reinforce why behavioral changes are necessary. This type of "learning" is attitudinal in nature, and often presents the biggest challenges.

5. **Learning occurs best when an opportunity is provided to apply the information or skills immediately.** Following a client-teaching session, the nurse allocates time for "doing." This may include encouraging the client to handle equipment, ask questions, or clarify procedural steps. A lapse of too much time between explanation

and application of knowledge can hinder learning. The teacher should provide ample time for the learner to practice and refine the technique of a new skill.

If nurses are to assess patients, adapt content and methods, and evaluate effectiveness, they must have the knowledge and skills to do so. They must also be able to effectively use the knowledge and skills within the limited time frames they have to teach patients and their caregivers. The nurse's role is to think critically about clients and their circumstances in order to create a learning opportunity for the patient that promotes safety and optimizes independence. Questions the nurse considers prior to carrying out a teaching plan for the client include:

1. Is the client (and/or caregiver) able to demonstrate the behavior safely and independently?

2. What knowledge and skills must the nurse possess or develop to become more effective?

3. What can the nurse do to integrate basic teaching principles into practice to promote the client's health, safety, and independence?

A TEAM APPROACH

Client-teaching plans often break down because of a lack of individualized client assessment. A "one-size-fits-all" approach fails to consider factors that include but are not limited to the individual's physical status, environment, pain status, emotional state, cognitive level, and readiness to learn. It is impossible for the nurse to gather all of this information during an initial admission assessment. Crucial to an effective teaching plan is the input of other members of the health care team (physicians, physical therapists, case management personnel) to add to assessment data and to communicate consistently.

LEARNING STYLES

Kolb (1984) developed a framework for identifying an individual's learning style, suggesting that learning is a process as well as an outcome. This model involves four stages associated with distinct learning styles: *diverging* concerns people who would rather "watch" than "do," gathering information and using imagination to solve problems; *assimilating* is a concise, logical approach where individuals prefer readings and lectures, and to explore analytical models; *converging* involves those who enjoy experimenting with new ideas; and *accommodating* is when learners prefer to take a practical, experiential approach, working in teams to complete tasks.

Kolb's theory provides a rationale for a variety of learning methods. These methods involve learning by doing, independent, and work and problem-based learning. If learning is to be consolidated and implemented in practice, these components must be included (Frankel, 2009).

Another model to consider when assessing learning styles is the Visual–Auditory–Kinesthetic/Tactile (VAK/T) Questionnaire (Chislett & Chapman, 2005). This instrument suggests that preferred learning style is determined by a person's dominant use of one of the three sensory receivers.

Visual learners prefer to see and to read. Seeing and reading are important for visual learners. Linguistic visual learners learn through use of the written word. Computer-based instruction, books, and articles are examples of linguistic visual learning tools. Spatial visual learners favor pictures, models, and demonstrations.

Auditory learners prefer speaking and listening. Examples include discussion, hearing directions, expert lectures, audiotapes, repeating and hearing information repeated out loud, and repeating information to themselves. The learners with auditory learning style like to hear detailed directions and learn things one at a time. Auditory learners benefit from listening to a talk and participating in discussions.

Kinesthetic learners prefer touch and movement. These individuals learn best by "hands on" activities, writing and rewriting material, interacting with the written word, drawing pictures, and moving while learning. These learners like to be involved with physical experiences; touching, feeling, holding, doing, and practical hands-on experiences.

Before actually carrying out a teaching session, the nurse may ask the client how he or she learns best: "What's the first thing you do when you need to learn something new?" As a preliminary step in planning a teaching session, a question such as this can provide valuable insight into how a client best learns.

HEALTH LITERACY

A critical issue for health care providers is that of health literacy, "the client's ability to obtain, process, and understand basic health information and services needed to make appropriate health decisions and follow

instructions for treatment" (Institute of Medicine [IOM], 2004). It is important for nurses to recognize indications that the client's ability to assimi-
late basic health information may be in jeopardy. "Red flags" (McNeill,
2012, p. 3) suggest a possible concern with learning health information.
This should inform the nurse to examine the situation and to intervene
appropriately.

"Red flags" include "forgotten" glasses that prevent patients from
reading printed instructions or forms, missed appointments due to naviga-
tion problems or lack of understanding of directions, difficulty completing
health forms, inability to list and describe the purpose of prescribed medications, limited questioning of the health care provider, and apparent lack
of follow-through on self-care instructions (Fernandez & Schillinger, 2009;
Katz, Jacobson, Veledar, & Kripalani, 2007).

Chew et al. have developed three specific screening questions that have
been shown to identify clients with low levels of health literacy (Chew,
Bradley, & Boyko, 2004). Employing a five-point Likert scale, the questions
ask: "How confident are you in filling out medical forms by yourself?"
("Not at all Confident" to "Very Confident" response); "How often do you
have someone help you read hospital materials?" ("Always" to "Never"
response); and "How often do you have problems learning about your
medical condition because of difficulty understanding written information?" ("Always" to "Never" response).

Although Chew et al.'s three questions are effective in identifying patients
having low health literacy, they may miss clients' compensatory behaviors
when misunderstanding instructions. Without these assessment data, it is
difficult for health professionals to either support patients in using compensatory behaviors that will promote understanding or to suggest behaviors
that would better help patients understand vital health information.

McNeil (2012) states that asking "What do you want to know first?"
(p. 4) helps the nurse understand the client's most pressing concern.
Addressing this directly alleviates anxiety and expedites learning needs;
from there, client and nurse can move on to other matters. Moreover, the
question demonstrates that the nurse cares about the client as an individual.
This creates an environment conducive to learning, and, ultimately, the client as active participant in the plan of care.

Following clarification regarding client needs, the nurse can then formulate individualized objectives in consideration of what the client should
be able to *demonstrate, verbalize,* or *perform* after the education is provided:
"By ____(date), the client states the signs and symptoms of hypoglycemia."

Written objectives speak to the three domains of learning, using Bloom's Taxonomy (Anderson et al., 2000):

- *Cognitive ("Head")* addresses changes in knowledge: "Upon discharge, the client identifies three symptoms that would require alerting her physician."
- *Affective ("Heart")* involves those changes in attitude that will affect compliance: "Following the teaching session, the client verbalizes the effects his smoking has not only on his health, but the well-being of his wife and children."
- *Psychomotor ("Hands")* entails changes in the ability to perform a task: "At the end of this teaching session, the client demonstrates appropriate self-injection technique with the administration of insulin."

EVALUATION OF CLIENT LEARNING

After an assessment has been completed, expected outcomes have been identified, objectives have been developed, and adult learning principles have been utilized, how does the nurse evaluate the patient's ability to do what must be done in order to be safe?

The "teach-back" or "show me" method (Xu, 2012) is the process of asking clients to repeat in their own words what they need to know or do. One of the easiest ways to close any communication gaps, the nurse observes the client actually return-demonstrate a skill. This provides an opportunity to assess for understanding and, if necessary, reteach the information. Additionally, it assists the nurse in determining the explanations and communication strategies that are most commonly understood by patients. With the increasing incidence of chronic disease, patient self-management has become more important. Incorporating the teach-back method into your daily practice can improve client knowledge and self-management skills.

STRATEGIES FOR INCORPORATING TEACHING IN DAILY NURSING PRACTICE

Timing. Timing is crucial when it comes to learning. Clients who have just received critical news or a serious diagnosis will need time to cope with associated feelings of grief, powerlessness, fear, and vulnerability. These emotions can severely impair the ability to learn. Evaluate readiness to learn and plan with the client the optimal time for teaching. Delivering somewhat complex information should be done in segments, not packed in all at once on the day of discharge. It is not appropriate to crowd all the patient teaching into the day of discharge. Look for teachable moments during the day, avoiding visiting hours or meal times.

Emphasize the Basics. It is important to consider the educational level of the patient when teaching. Some patients might be illiterate and may not be able to read handouts, or they might not be able to understand complex medical jargon. To avoid overwhelming the client, clearly define realistic goals and objectives. Before beginning teaching, both nurse and client should sit down together to discuss these goals and objectives. The significance of each goal should be clearly defined to the client for better understanding. Evaluate these goals on a continuous basis.

Sensory Awareness. Assess the client's vision and hearing abilities. Does the client wear glasses, contacts, or hearing aids? Are they with the client in the hospital? Are they in good repair?

Additionally, consideration of pain and pain control is vital before a teaching plan can be put into effect. Evaluate the client's pain level using selected measurement tools (e.g., 0–10 pain scale), evaluate the effectiveness of the selected pain medication, and assess if (and which) nonpharmacological methods for pain relief (massage, guided imagery, breathing and relaxation exercises) have been used in the past.

Cost Factors. For many clients, cost is a major factor in compliance with care. It may not be practical to recommend that they join a fitness center as a means of weight reduction. Whether it be endorsing purchase of a glucometer for the diabetic client or a scale for the dialysis client, it is important to consider the cost of equipment.

Documentation. Whenever teaching a new skill, nursing documentation is important. If the client has difficulty with a certain skill or needs special assistance with equipment, this should be documented so that accommodations or further instruction can be provided. Also, documentation guides the oncoming nurse in planning client care by affording him or her the opportunity to see what teaching has been carried out and which topics need reinforcement and attention.

SAMPLE CASE STUDY AND TEACHING PLAN

Background

DK is a 58-year-old female client brought by ambulance to the emergency department in diabetic ketoacidosis. Her symptoms upon admission included confusion, lethargy, fatigue, polydipsia, and polyuria. Her blood sugar was 620 mg/dL. A newly diagnosed diabetic, DK was admitted to the intensive care unit for 3 days before being transferred to the telemetry unit for continued treatment and teaching. Additionally, she is being prepared for a colonoscopy due to a suspicious area noted on her cecum during an abdominal ultrasound.

Past Medical History

Hypertension, depression, hypothyroidism, deep vein thrombosis, arthritis.

Assessment of Learner/Readiness to Learn

DK is alert and oriented to person, place, and time. She denies any pain and appears physically comfortable. She ambulates independently. She speaks and reads English. She is divorced and lives at home with her adult children. She wears glasses. She states her vision is blurry at times, which is new to her and related to this hospitalization. She has difficulty with fine motor coordination due to arthritis in her hands. She is left-handed. DK expresses doubts about being able to draw insulin into a syringe correctly. She is beginning to ask questions about proper diet choices. She has mentioned that she goes to the bakery shop next door to her home every day and doesn't want to "give that up." She is also asking questions about diabetes. She is concerned about her upcoming colonoscopy. At times she appears worried about her situation; when family is present she appears confident. Family members visit daily and include two daughters and a son with Down's syndrome. When alone with the nurse, she expresses concern about the stresses of her adult children and grandchildren depending on her.

Nursing Diagnoses

- Deficient knowledge related to unfamiliarity with information resources secondary to new diagnosis of diabetes mellitus as evidenced by inaccurate performance of test (Ackley & Ladwig, 2011, p. 517).
- Ineffective coping related to inadequate opportunity to prepare for stressor secondary to new diagnosis of diabetes mellitus as evidenced by fatigue (Ackley & Ladwig, 2011, p. 294).

Expected Learning Outcomes

By the end of the second day of teaching, the client will:

1. Demonstrate the appropriate technique for checking blood sugar.
2. Demonstrate proper technique for drawing correct insulin dose into a syringe.
3. Demonstrate proper technique for self-administration of insulin.
4. Verbalize signs and symptoms of hypo- and hyperglycemia.

Content

1. Demonstrate checking blood sugar: Assemble supplies: glucometer, test strips, lancets, and notebook for tracking results. Wash hands. Turn on glucometer and check battery level. Insert a test strip into glucometer. Obtain blood sample by pressing lancet against the side of the fingertip, avoiding the sensitive finger pad. Apply drop of blood to test strip. Do not squeeze the finger to obtain blood; if necessary, hold the hand down for a few minutes just prior to using the lancet. Apply pressure to the site to promote clotting. Record results in a notebook. Also make note of any signs of hypo- or hyperglycemia at the time. Discard used lancet and test strip. Check blood sugar four times a day—before meals and at bedtime, or as prescribed.
2. Demonstrate drawing dose of insulin into syringe: Practice materials provided include an insulin syringe, alcohol swabs, and 10 mL vial of normal saline for patient to begin learning how to draw up a liquid

into a syringe. Determine dose of insulin needed according to doctor's orders. Insulin is a medication that is given in "units." Assemble the materials needed: insulin vial, insulin syringe, and alcohol swab. Clean the top of the insulin vial with an alcohol swab and let dry. Remove the cap of the syringe and, using the dominant (left) hand, insert it into the insulin vial. In the nondominant (right) hand, holding the vial and syringe in a straight line, tip them upside down so the vial is above the syringe. Hold vial and syringe at eye level. Pull down on the plunger of the syringe with the left hand, to draw out the proper number of units to be given. Keeping vial and syringe in a straight line, pull the needle out of the vial.

3. Demonstrate administering insulin injection: Determine location to give injection. It should be injected into the layer of fat just below the surface of the skin. Sites used include the abdomen (at least 1 inch away from the umbilicus), thigh, and upper arm. Clean/swab the area, pinch an area of skin with the nondominant (right) hand, push the needle into the skin to the hub, release the skin with the right hand, and press down on the plunger to deliver the dose.

4. Remove the needle and retract/use safety cover. Discard needle in a safe place, away from children, and store insulin vial according to directions.

5. Verbalize signs of hypoglycemia and hyperglycemia: A normal blood sugar reading is between 70 mg/dL and 110 mg/dL. If blood sugar is below 70 mg/dL, it is too low; this is called hypoglycemia. Signs of hypoglycemia include hunger, nervousness, shakiness, dizziness, lightheadedness, perspiring, sleepiness, and confusion. These can progress to unconsciousness. Reasons for a low blood sugar include skipping a meal, taking too much insulin, and illness. If you experience these feelings, check your blood sugar right away and have some sugar, such as a glass of juice or a glucose tablet. An injection of glucagon may be needed. Seek medical attention/call 911 if symptoms are severe, before confusion sets in. If your blood sugar is too high, this is called hyperglycemia. Signs of this include increased thirst, hunger, frequent urination, blurred vision, dry mouth, and sleepiness/fatigue. It can progress to stupor and coma. Reasons for hyperglycemia include eating too many carbohydrates, infection, illness, stress, certain medications such as prednisone, and decreasing

the amount of exercise. If you experience these signs, check your blood sugar right away. Take insulin as directed. Try to maintain good nutrition and exercise habits. Contact your doctor or call 911 in an emergency (New, 2010).

Teaching Methods

The nurse will:

1. Plan teaching session, including setting learning goal with client ahead of time; gathering supplies for demonstrations; and providing a quiet, well-lit learning environment free of distractions. The client will need to have her glasses present. Address short-term goals first, such as checking blood sugar and giving insulin.
2. Describe and demonstrate proper method for checking blood sugar.
3. Describe and demonstrate proper method for drawing dose of insulin.
4. Describe and demonstrate proper method for injecting insulin.
5. Discuss signs of hypo- and hyperglycemia.
6. Discuss healthy food choices.

Evaluation

1. The patient demonstrated proper technique for checking her blood sugar, drawing insulin, and injecting herself, but she needed cueing throughout the process. Patient will need further teaching, practice, and reinforcement to master the tasks. She expresses the feeling, "I don't know if I can do this." Patient will need further teaching with nurses and diabetes nurse practitioner prior to discharge.
2. The patient was unable to list signs of hypo- and hyperglycemia. Further teaching and handouts will be needed.
3. The patient is beginning to discuss food choices. She chose a garden salad with lettuce, vegetables, and grilled chicken for dinner. She would benefit from further teaching and support from the dietician prior to discharge.

CHAPTER 5 REFLECTIVE QUESTIONS

1. In your practice setting, how do you begin to assess the learning needs of your organization's client population?

2. If teaching clients is a health care team approach in your practice setting, how do you guarantee consistency in the delivery of educational content? What problems might occur with inconsistencies in teaching? How might your team address this issue?

3. Think back to your most effective teaching session with a client. To what do you attribute this success? Why?

4. How would you describe your individual teaching style?

CHAPTER 6

Cultural Considerations in Nursing

OBJECTIVES

1. Define the concepts of culture relevant to health and health-seeking behaviors.
2. Recognize strategies to broaden the cultural and ethnic diversity in nursing.
3. Identify current barriers to health care in society.
4. Discuss components of culture pertinent to nursing care.
5. Discuss the following concepts related to diversity:
   a. Multiculturalism
   b. Cultural sensitivity
   c. Ethnocentrism

KEY TERMS

Cultural sensitivity

Diversity

Ethnocentrism

Kleinman assessment questions

Multiculturalism

Transcultural nursing

STANDARDS

Patient-Centered Care		
Definition: Recognize the patient or designee as the source of control and full partner in providing compassionate and coordinated care based on respect for patient's preferences, values, and needs.		
Knowledge	Skills	Attitudes
Integrate understanding of multiple dimensions of patient-centered care: • patient/family/community preferences, values • coordination and integration of care • information, communication, and education • physical comfort and emotional support • involvement of family and friends • transition and continuity Describe how diverse cultural, ethnic, and social backgrounds function as sources of patient, family, and community values	Elicit patient values, preferences, and expressed needs as part of clinical interview, implementation of care plan, and evaluation of care. Communicate patient values, preferences, and expressed needs to other members of health care team Provide patient-centered care with sensitivity and respect for the diversity of human experience	Value seeing health care situations "through patients' eyes." Respect and encourage individual expression of patient values, preferences, and expressed needs Value the patient's expertise with own health and symptoms Seek learning opportunities with patients who represent all aspects of human diversity. Recognize personally held attitudes about working with patients from different ethnic, cultural, and social backgrounds. Willingly support patient-centered care for individuals and groups whose values differ from own

To care for someone, I must know who I am.
To care for someone, I must know who the other is.
To care for someone, I must be able to bridge the gap
between myself and the other.

Nurse Theorist Jean Watson

NO CURE WITHOUT CARING

Many years ago, as a novice LPN, I heard the phrase "no cure without caring." I remember having several patients in my clinical experiences in nursing school who spoke different languages and who were not native to America. On many occasions it made a difference on how many people we allowed in the room. For a new mother from Africa, it meant for her to have 10 people (adults and children) in the room with her for the entire day. For others I took care of, it meant sometimes just having a reliable translator. For an older Italian man, it meant having his Italian, non-English speaking lady friend care for all of his personal care other than medication or treatments. I find it so interesting to meet people with different customs. We care for them, but they teach us so much more.

Nursing student

This chapter introduces the student to nursing in a culturally diverse world. Nurses need to become informed about and sensitive to culturally diverse subjective meanings of health, illness, caring, and healing practice. A transcultural caring perspective is considered essential for nurses in order to deliver quality health care to all clients.

Culture shapes language, behaviors, values, and institutions. Understanding culture can help nurses develop knowledge of how to interact with other groups and avoid prejudice, stereotypes, and biases. To be culturally sensitive means to understand how clients present themselves based on their culture. Cultural awareness can assist the nurse in ensuring the delivery of care that is informed, effective, and respectful for all clients.

TRANSCULTURAL NURSING

As health professionals living in a multicultural society, nurses interact with and care for individuals who are culturally and ethnically different from themselves. At times, any barriers are easily crossed, with clear recognition of clients' core values and beliefs. At other times, the barrier is more difficult to penetrate. Even with the assistance of an interpreter, communication difficulties arise.

Narayanasamy (2002) developed the ACCESS model in order to help health professionals bridge the cultural gap and provide acceptable transcultural care:

Assessment: Focus on the cultural aspects of the client's lifestyle, health beliefs, and health practices.

Communication: Be aware of variations in verbal and nonverbal responses.

Cultural negotiation and compromise: Develop a heightened awareness of aspects of other people's culture.

Establishing respect and rapport: Create a therapeutic relationship that conveys genuine respect for the client's cultural beliefs and values.

Sensitivity: Deliver culturally sensitive care to a culturally diverse group.

Safety: Enable clients to derive a sense of cultural safety.

Clients benefit when nurses learn more about and become confident in their ability to care for diverse cultural groups. Specifically, clients may be more satisfied with their health care interactions and may increase treatment compliance. Nurses have many ways to intervene with patients in a culturally appropriate way. However, nurses must be aware of the factors that affect their ability to provide culturally sensitive care, particularly if their biases are unconscious. Factors that negatively impact cultural competence and delivery of culturally competent care include ethnocentrism (the belief in superiority of one's ethnic group), essentialism (viewing other groups as essentially different), and power differences (the power imbalance in the patient–provider relationship).

MULTICULTURALISM

It is not our differences that divide us. It is our inability to recognize, accept, and celebrate those differences.

Audre Lorde

To Leininger and McFarland (2002), multiculturalism refers to the viewpoint that there are many diverse cultures and subcultures in the world that need to be recognized, valued, and understood for their differences and similarities. Multiculturalism is often linked with transcultural nursing in focusing on comparative differences and similarities among cultures in relation to humanistic care, health, wellness, illness, healing patterns, beliefs, and values. Gustafson (2005) defined transcultural nursing as "the humanistic and scientific study of all people from different cultures in the world with thought to the ways the nurse can assist people with their daily health and living needs" (p. 4). Providing culture-specific and universal nursing care practices is essential not only for the clients' health but when dealing with adverse human conditions, illness, or death in culturally meaningful ways.

A multicultural or transcultural focus makes nurses think about differences and similarities among people regarding their special needs and concerns to develop different ways to assist clients. As nurses discover the client's particular cultural beliefs and values, they learn ways to provide sensitive, compassionate, and competent care that is beneficial and satisfying to the client (Leininger & McFarland, 2002).

CULTURAL SENSITIVITY

We are different so that we can know our need of one another, for no one is ultimately self-sufficient. A completely self-sufficient person would be subhuman.

Archbishop Desmond Tutu
Civil rights activist, Nobel Laureate

With rising globalization leading to a substantial growth in immigration, there is a significant need for nurses to deliver culturally sensitive care to expanding, diverse client groups. However, the inability to meet the need to provide care to minority populations has contributed to disparities in health and health care (McHenry, 2007). A lack of understanding of cultural health values and the perpetuation of ethnocentric Western values explains the racial patterns in the use of the health services. Evidence from Spain, the United States, Canada, and the Netherlands demonstrates that the use of health services is lower in immigrant groups when compared to their nonimmigrant counterparts (Chambers, Thompson, & Narayanasamy, 2013).

Leininger and McFarland (2006) provided the first formal definition of transcultural nursing and health–illness practices, beliefs, and values.

According to this definition, cultural competence is demonstrated when practitioners understand and appreciate differences in health beliefs and behaviors, recognize and respect variations that occur within cultural groups, and are able to adjust their practice to provide effective interventions for people from various cultures.

To provide culturally congruent care that benefits, satisfies, and is meaningful to the clients nurses serve, Leininger and McFarland (1991) conceptualize three major modes to guide nursing judgments, decisions, and actions: cultural care preservation and/or maintenance, where the nurse complies with the client's cultural practices that have worked well in the past; cultural care accommodation and/or negotiation, where the nurse accommodates the client's treatment, food, or religious practices; and care repatterning or restructuring, where the nurse develops ways to restructure care to meet the client's cultural needs (p. 41).

How can nurses develop cultural awareness? What skills do nurses need to provide culturally sensitive care, specifically relating to patient education? The fundamental communication skills of listening, observation, empathy, and individualized therapeutic responses (as in patient-centered care) are not new to nurses.

The Kleinman questions (Kleinman, Eisenberg, & Good, 1978) apply therapeutic communication skills in order to assess the client's cultural needs. The following eight questions were designed to assist the health care provider when interviewing clients from diverse cultures. In this way, the provider does not need to know the specifics of the culture beforehand; instead, he or she can specifically find out how that culture is reflected in the expression and understanding of the symptoms and illness presented by the client.

1. What do you think caused the problem?
2. Why do you think it happened when it did?
3. What do you think your sickness does to you? How does it work?
4. How severe is your sickness? Will it have a short course?
5. What kind of treatment do you think you should receive?
6. What are the most important results you hope to receive from this treatment?
7. What are the chief problems your sickness has caused for you?
8. What do you fear most about your sickness?
   (Kleinman et al., 1978, p. 256)

Once the nurse perceives how the client views the illness, it becomes much easier to individualize care. Information, treatments, and education relating to self-care skills can then be presented within the client's framework. This client-centered approach demonstrates respect and minimizes possible misinterpretation of the facts.

The Kleinman questions are open-ended and can be incorporated into conversation, the admission interview, and early on in the admission process, as needed. These questions are appropriate for all patients. However, if English is not the patient's primary language, the interviewer should consider using an interpreter. In this way, the client's cultural views are better communicated in the language of the culture.

Kleinman encourages the interviewer to "listen deeply to the responses, without judgment" (p. 257) in order to correctly understand the patient's viewpoint. If the client is from a different culture, religion, or socioeconomic group, the interviewer may not accurately anticipate what he or she will hear. Ask for clarification or detail as necessary and appropriate.

Acknowledge that some questions may not be appropriate for all clients. If asked "What kind of treatment do you think you should receive?" the client may reply, "Why are you asking me? That's up to the doctor! Doesn't he know what he's doing?" Respond to a reaction such as this with a statement explaining that some clients come with an idea that they need a particular treatment. Additionally, document and report pertinent client assessment findings for consistency and accuracy of communication with other members of the health care team.

Sharing stories may also provide concrete examples of interactions with clients from diverse cultures. A poignant example is found in author Anne Fadiman's (1997) work, *The Spirit Catches You and You Fall Down: A Hmong Child, Her American Doctors, and the Collision of Two Cultures.* This book describes in detail the continual misunderstandings, errors, and gaps in care due to miscommunication between health care providers and the family of a chronically ill Hmong child.

The primary purposes of client education are to ensure informed consent and to promote self-care skills that improve health outcomes. In client-centered care, the clients themselves are viewed as experts in their life experiences relating to health. They are respected as knowledgeable partners. In this model, health care providers and clients negotiate, collaborate, and together develop a plan of care. When interventions are tailored to the client and with the client, many of the challenges that create noncompliance are eliminated.

Using the eight assessment questions involves both nurse and client right from the admission process. Developing cultural sensitivity and cultural awareness, however, is a work in progress, with careful attention to listening, observation, and empathy skills. Evidence obtained must be considered in light of the client's concerns and preferences (Melnyk & Fineout-Overholt, 2010).

The one way to move from a theoretical transcultural framework to the functional provision of culturally responsible client care is to perform it (London, 2008). This client-centered approach paves the way for the nurse to enter into the relationship without preconceived notions or misinformation of the client's culture. Coupled with this is the recommendation that reflection on one's own judgments, agenda setting, and social practices in comparison to those of clients from other cultural groups can help bridge the gap between ethnocentric and culturally sensitive care (Chambers et al., 2013).

ORGANIZATIONS INVESTED IN FOSTERING CULTURAL AWARENESS

In 1991, the American Nurses Association (ANA) acknowledged culture as "one of the organizing concepts upon which nursing is cased and defined" (p.1). In 2008, the American Association of Colleges of Nursing (2008a) identified five competencies essential for baccalaureate-prepared nurses:

1. Apply knowledge of social and cultural factors that affect nursing and health care across multiple contexts.
2. Use relevant data sources and best evidence in providing culturally competent care.
3. Promote achievement of safe and quality outcomes of care for diverse populations.
4. Advocate for social justice, including commitment to the health of vulnerable populations and the elimination of health disparities.
5. Participate in continuous cultural competence development.

Both The Joint Commission and the National Committee for Quality Assurance have encouraged health care professionals to recognize and respect cultural differences (Levine, 2012). In response to these reports, health care organizations have introduced "interactive client engagement technology" into their client education programs, providing services in several languages. These responses exemplify that as nursing focuses more on culture and cultural practices, outcomes reflect a shift in a positive direction (Levine, 2012).

In her transcultural nursing research, Leininger advanced nursing's understanding of cultural context. Cultural competence is defined as the ability to interact appropriately with others through cultural understanding and is an expectation of the health care professional; however, nurses should be sensitive to the difference between "learning of" and "learning from" another culture (Masters, 2014, p. 135).

CHAPTER 6 REFLECTIVE QUESTIONS

Continually reflecting on your reactions to the cultures of your clients will assist you in providing culturally acceptable care.

1. How would you define values clarification? How would you interpret its usefulness in understanding cultures?

2. What would you describe as your culture?

3. Reflect on an occasion when you were with a group of people from another country. What were the similarities and differences in culture?

4. How would you rank the following in order of importance: ethnicity, family, work, diet, and religion? Do you believe that your clients have the same priorities?

5. How might a client from another culture interpret your body language (posture, eye contact, tone of your voice)?

PART III

Role Competencies
for the
Baccalaureate-Prepared Nurse

CHAPTER 7

Leadership and Management

OBJECTIVES

1. Contrast leadership and management roles and responsibilities.
2. Discuss the attainment of leadership skills.
3. Examine managing the business of leadership.
4. Compare different leadership and management styles.
5. Identify the qualities of a transformational leader.
6. Describe shared governance as a model for collaborative decision making.

KEY TERMS

Affiliative	Leadership
Authoritarian	Management
Conflict resolution	Permissive
Democratic	Transactional
Incivility	Transformational

STANDARDS

Teamwork and Collaboration		
Definition: Function effectively within nursing and interprofessional teams, fostering open communication, mutual respect, and shared decision making to achieve quality patient care.		
Knowledge	**Skills**	**Attitudes**
Describe own strengths, limitations, and values in functioning as a member of a team	Demonstrate awareness of own strengths and limitations as a team member. Initiate plan for self-development as a team member Act with integrity, consistency, and respect for differing views	Acknowledge own potential to contribute to effective team functioning. Appreciate importance of intra- and inter-professional collaboration
Describe scopes of practice and roles of health care team members. Describe strategies for identifying and managing overlaps in team member roles and accountabilities Recognize contributions of other individuals and groups in helping patient/family achieve health goals	Function competently within own scope of practice as a member of the health care team. Assume role of team member or leader based on the situation Initiate requests for help when appropriate to situation Clarify roles and accountabilities under conditions of potential overlap in team member functioning. Integrate the contributions of others who play a role in helping patient/family achieve health goals	Value the perspectives and expertise of all health team members. Respect the centrality of the patient/family as core members of any health care team Respect the unique attributes that members bring to a team, including variations in professional orientations and accountabilities

(continued)

Knowledge	Skills	Attitudes
Analyze differences in communication-style preferences among patients and families, nurses, and other members of the health team. Describe impact of own communication style on others. Discuss effective strategies for communicating and resolving conflict	Communicate with team members, adapting own style of communicating to needs of the team and situation. Demonstrate commitment to team goals Solicit input from other team members to improve individual, as well as team, performance Initiate actions to resolve conflict	Value teamwork and the relationships upon which it is based. Value different styles of communication used by patients, families, and health care providers Contribute to resolution of conflict and disagreement
Describe examples of the impact of team functioning on safety and quality of care. Explain how authority gradients influence team-work and patient safety	Follow communication practices that minimize risks associated with handoffs among providers and across transitions in care. Assert own position/ perspective in discussions about patient care. Choose communication styles that diminish the risks associated with authority gradients among team members	Appreciate the risks associated with handoffs among providers and across transitions in care
Identify system barriers and facilitators of effective team functioning. Examine strategies for improving systems to support team functioning	Participate in designing systems that support effective teamwork	Value the influence of system solutions in achieving effective team functioning

L eadership and management skills are the responsibility of all professional nurses. Knowledge of the different, yet linked, roles of leader
and manager is fundamental to every nurse's ability to work within the
health care system. As individual, family, and community advocates and
leaders, nurses offer a wide variety of support, resources, and services.

In this chapter, the terms leadership and management are described
and differentiated, and the role of the baccalaureate-prepared nurse as
leader and manager is explored. Effective leadership is a learned process involving an understanding of the needs and goals that motivate
individuals, coupled with the interpersonal skills to influence them.
Management involves planning, organizing, leading, delegating, controlling, and power. The degree to which a nurse carries out these functions
depends on the position the nurse holds in the organization; regardless
of position, however, authority and accountability remain important to
the process.

Christmas (2009) states that leadership skills are required at every level
in the nursing profession, and that nurses display leadership roles when
making daily decisions about client care: "True leadership requires equal
parts vision and humility, with the ability to confront hard truths and to
coach and mentor" (p. 133).

TITLE DOESN'T MATTER

*I am an LPN fortunate enough to work in the ER. We use a team
approach whenever a new client arrives; whoever is free comes into
the room and assists with getting the individual settled. The local fire
department calls in to report they are on their way with a "34-year-old
female, 5 months pregnant, status postseizure." They arrive about
10 minutes later. In the exam room, the patient shouts "I can't
breathe!" She is 26 weeks pregnant and her husband is at home
with their two other young children. We are taking vital signs when
her eyes roll back in her head and she goes into respiratory arrest.
Somebody shouts "Call a code!" The code cart is wheeled into the
room and the physician intubates her. He no sooner asked for the
neonatologists and OB-GYN physicians to be paged to come to the ER
when the patient goes into cardiac arrest. CPR is initiated immediately. Within a matter of seconds the decision to deliver the baby is
made. While CPR is being performed, the OB surgeon performs an
emergency cesarean section. The lifeless baby that fits in the palm of*

his hand is intubated and taken to NICU. We are still doing CPR on the mother, which is difficult, as the surgeon is trying to quickly close the incision. My hands are slipping on blood and betadine. I remember once asking the doctor if I should stop for a minute so he could finish, and he told me to keep going. After what seemed like forever, we got pulses back.

We then had the task of transferring the patient out during a raging blizzard. An ambulance transfers the patient to the cath lab with two of our nurses and our ER doctor. She was found to have two massive pulmonary emboli. She experienced cardiac arrest a second time in the cath lab; fortunately, they were able to regain pulses, and she was stabilized.

Next week we will be celebrating the baby's first birthday, with her mother, father, and older siblings. Everyone who was involved with this case will be there to celebrate not one, but two, miracles. On that particular day, everything fell into place perfectly. If you were in that room, involved in the care of both patients, it didn't matter what your title was, all that mattered was that we accomplished the outcome that we did.

Delegation and leadership skills, professional communication with confidence, as well as expanding on previously gained nursing knowledge are three areas I would like to improve on as I return to school for my bachelor's degree in nursing. Feeling more confident in professional communication abilities I think could help with leadership, and eventually being able to step into the role of a nurse manager.

Nursing student

DIFFERENTIATING LEADERSHIP AND MANAGEMENT

Although leadership and management roles are different, the terms "leader" and "manager" are often used interchangeably. Leadership is defined as the "process of influencing people to accomplish goals" (Huber, 2006, p. 7). A leader seeks input and collaborates with all members of the team, guiding them toward mutually agreed-upon goals. Management involves not only leadership but also "coordination and integration of resources through planning, organizing, coordinating, directing, and controlling to accomplish specific institutional goals and objectives" (Huber, 2006, p. 7). A manager values individuals' needs while planning the tasks to accomplish the team's goals. The nurse may be a leader or manager in the care of the individual client, the client's family, groups of clients, or the community.

Regardless of the setting, the nurse must demonstrate leadership and management skills in interacting with clients and their families and with nursing colleagues (Sherman & Pross, 2010).

The "power" that the leader has acquired has come informally from others in the group. Leaders focus on empowering as well as motivating, inspiring, and influencing others. True leaders must be sincere and energetic. A leader may be a risk-taker, but not to the extent that others feel that they are reckless.

Managers typically have an assigned position within the formal organization. A manager is expected to carry out specific duties and has definite responsibilities. Control over processes, decision making, and the work of others are included in the manager's role. Competent nursing managers are adept at coordinating resources, following rules, and meeting the goals and objectives of the organization. Control is a key element of the role. The contemporary view is that the manager focuses on planning, monitoring results, decision making, decision analysis, resource control, and development.

Kearney-Nunnery (2008) states that "a manager focuses on directing the group to meet the desired outcomes for the organization through thoughtful and careful planning, direction, monitoring recognition, development and representation" (p. 216), a characterization incorporating the human relationship component of the management role. Success in nursing management implies that the manager must be results oriented. However, the caution here is to not lose sight of the human interaction needed for a collaborative working environment. Kerfoot (2008) addresses this challenge in his explanation that a leader serves those under his guidance "first in order that they may serve their customers better because they are skilled and fulfilled human beings" (p. 134).

All nurses are leaders and managers at some level. The rapid and dramatic changes in health care make these skills more important than ever. Critical thinking, active listening, and coping skills are essential at all levels in today's nursing workforce. Effective leaders and managers see the future and lead the way toward a productive and efficient unit with workers that are satisfied and motivated. This can be accomplished through seeking out additional professional growth and learning opportunities, becoming politically aware and active, reading professional journals, and attending continuing education offerings relevant to nursing practice. No formal title of manager is required for these activities; a competent nursing leader and manager will take advantage of these and other opportunities.

LEADERSHIP SKILLS

One of the most decisive functions of leadership is the creation, management, and when necessary, the destruction and rebuilding of culture.

Edgar Schein
Organizational behavior and culture pioneer

There is no disagreement that a positive work environment is associated with job satisfaction, employee retention, improved patient outcomes, and organizational performance (Aiken, Havens, & Sloane, 2009). The American Nurses Credentialing Center (2013) credits positive work environments to a practice culture of communication, accountability, and collaboration; the existence of sufficient numbers of qualified nurses and nurse leaders; shared decision making at all levels; continued growth and development; and acknowledgment of the value of nursing's contributions.

Creating a healthy work environment requires strong nursing leadership at all levels of the organization. This is evident on clinical units where most front-line staff work and where patient care is delivered. If such a setting is to be realized, nurses in these roles will need guidance to develop the leadership skills needed to support such an endeavor. Leaders can ensure this by involving staff in the development of shared values in their work. Accessible nursing leaders play a key role in helping to give nurses a voice in improvement of the patient care environment. This requires a transition from a more traditional command-and-control style of staff supervision toward a transformational style of leadership (Shirey & Fisher, 2008).

Attainment of Magnet status through the American Nurses Credentialing Center is considered in nursing to be the gold standard for hospitals seeking to build healthy, supportive, and professional nursing practice environments (Drenkard, 2009). Outcomes show evidence that Magnet hospitals lead to patient and nurse satisfaction, enhanced recruitment and retention of nurses, and improved patient outcomes (Aiken et al., 2009; Stone & Gershan, 2009). Additionally, improvements in morbidity and mortality rates, failure-to-rescue rates, and patient safety were noted (Aiken et al., 2009; Armstrong, Laschinger, & Wong, 2009a, 2009b; Ulrich, Buerhaus, Donelan, Norman, & Dittus, 2009).

SHARED GOVERNANCE: COLLABORATIVE LEADERSHIP

Shared governance impacts client care by including nurses at all levels in organizational decision making regarding client care. Sullivan and Decker (2005) define shared governance as "an organizational paradigm based on the values of interdependence and accountability that allows nurses to make decisions in a decentralized environment" (p. 22). Designed to integrate those core values supported by professional practice, the shared governance model is aimed at improving the work setting, leading to job satisfaction and, ultimately, staff retention.

The focus of this model is to encourage nurses to participate in decision making at all levels of the organization. Nurses may join at their own request. Their role in shared governance may be included in their job description. Frequently, nurses participate by serving in decision-making groups, such as committees or task forces. The decisions they make may include working conditions, long-range planning, and productivity. The principal assumption of shared governance is that members of the organization will be committed to their organization's objectives if they have contributed in some way to goal planning and decision making.

In this model, the nurse manager becomes a consultant, teacher, and collaborator. In the managerial role, the nurse functions as a liaison for shared decision making between staff and administration. Shared governance is also a tool for "growing" nursing professionals. Participation in the shared governance model fosters professional growth behaviors that reflect a mature, collaborative decision maker and, ultimately, a future nursing leader.

CREATING LEADERS

Leadership skills begin with understanding one's self. Personal mastery is a critical component for leadership success. Outstanding leaders demonstrate self-confidence and are able to trust and empower others. They understand how their actions impact others and are perceptive to environmental cues. They develop an awareness of the importance of emotional intelligence in leadership. This authenticity in nursing leadership is viewed as the needed link to a healthy work environment. Becoming an authentic leader requires self-discovery, self-improvement, reflection, and renewal (Faila & Stichler, 2008).

The art of leadership involves managing relationships with others and influencing their behaviors. Guiding team members to get past day-to-day problems, conflicts, and communication issues and move toward the goals of working as a high-performance work team presents a significant leadership challenge for emerging leaders.

Leaders are urged to use briefings and debriefings in order to keep communication lines open (Sherman & Eggenberger, 2009). Even in the most ideal of environments, communication breakdown and conflict occur on teams. If managed effectively by emerging leaders, these situations can be seen as opportunities for learning and growth. Unresolved conflict can lead to loss of productivity, errors, client dissatisfaction, staff exodus, and an overall dysfunctional work environment.

Acknowledging staff members' work ethic and contributions to the position are an essential leadership obligation. Managing conflict well within a given environment fosters a culture where workers feel they are appreciated and their opinion is respected. Credit given for an individual's efforts fosters both professional and personal development. Such recognition can range from a leader's simple "thank you" at the end of a shift to recommendation of a staff member for a service award.

MANAGING THE BUSINESS OF LEADERSHIP

Health care reform discussions have focused on the cost of care in the United States, putting additional stress on leaders to run organizations more efficiently while grappling with the challenges of improving quality and client outcomes (Van Dyke, 2008). Despite the need to become more financially conscious, nurse leaders often find fiscal responsibility a daunting task. However, if nurses cannot comprehend the financial consequences and costs of decisions, they will be unsuccessful at securing the necessary resources to staff and manage units.

Nurse managers are in the unique position of involving rising leaders in the development and monitoring of a unit budget. For most units, staffing will be the single biggest budget item and area of concern. Leaders can be involved in analyzing staffing and productivity reports, as well as projects to review staffing variances and create staffing alternatives. With a trend toward hospital reimbursement for "nursing-sensitive" performance measures, emerging leaders must appreciate that nursing care outcomes affect the financial "bottom line" of their institutions (Stichler, 2008, p. 527).

Growing future nurse leaders requires both thoughtful preparation and purposeful action. It is important to ensure that nurses develop the skills and competencies that will be needed for success in leadership. The development of a healthy workplace environment responsive to the needs of a dynamic health care environment can be the legacy veteran leaders can pass on to those novices taking on the challenge. The most significant contribution today's leaders can make for the future is to develop their successors so that they will adapt, thrive, and continue to learn.

LEADERSHIP STYLES IN NURSING MANAGEMENT

The success of a leader is measured by the positive influential ability to motivate colleagues to reach the same goals of both the leader and the organization. An additional method of assessing a leader is by the leadership style used to direct staff. Leadership styles arise from leadership theories. The leadership style, characteristics, and role effectiveness that each leader must have are compared here. Performance improvement and transformational leadership can change a culture of noncompliant nursing staff to one that promotes performance excellence within an organization.

Democratic nurse leaders include their colleagues in goal setting and decision making, seeking their suggestions and feedback. They consider this information along with their own research and opinions. This leadership style also encourages the personal and professional development of nurses and allows them some autonomy. With its emphasis on individual nurses and their contributions to the team, this style often motivates employees to take initiative and consistently contribute their best efforts. The democratic style of leadership allows the employee to take part in goal setting and the decision-making process. Information or suggestions received from employees are taken into consideration and used when feasible. While allowing for input from employees, the final decision is made by the leader. However, when a particular area or topic is unfamiliar, the democratic leader is receptive to ideas and suggestions (Mills, 2007). Democratic leadership behaviors that enhance effectiveness include encouraging others to take part in the decision-making process; developing skills of employees; and encouraging team members to be in control of their own work. This motivates members of the team to work harder (Krause, 2007).

The *affiliative leadership style* puts the individual first. It accentuates the well-being and job satisfaction of team members. Affiliative leaders often take a passive approach to managing staff. They may hesitate to take a strong stance regarding decision making, but strive to ensure tasks are completed on time. The style recovers morale to a broken team, but can inhibit authority and may interfere with the leader's ability to step in when decisive action is required. Without a strong leader to guide the team's efforts, productivity and efficiency can also suffer. The behaviors associated with this style of leadership are a positive approach to employees, with a passive attitude. The leader here prefers not to anger team members, and often has difficulty when it comes to making a decision.

With a *transformational leadership style*, leaders encourage the personal and professional development of staff by endorsing teamwork, supporting self-esteem, and advising employees to participate in hospital policy and procedure committees. This style focuses on therapeutic communication skills, confidence, and integrity. Leaders use empathy to understand their employees' needs and motivations, tailoring their management and communication style to individual employees. Krause (2007) stated "the developmental nature of this style helps leaders achieve results by influencing, motivating, and inspiring employees over whom they may or may not have direct supervision" (p. 1).

In the *authoritarian leadership style*, some nurse managers prefer a stricter approach to leadership; they make all the decisions and rarely solicit input or feedback from employees. They issue orders and expect employees to carry them out promptly and without question. They also closely supervise employees, reducing the amount of staff autonomy. This leadership style allows for little innovation or flexibility; instead, it requires strict adherence to hospital policies. While this strategy often ensures tasks are completed quickly and efficiently, it can also cause discord and job dissatisfaction.

TRANSFORMATIONAL LEADERSHIP

A leader is best when people barely know he exists, when his work is done, his aim fulfilled, they will say: we did it ourselves.

Lao Tzu

Magnet designation is considered the gold standard of nursing practice excellence. In 2008, the American Nurses Credentialing Center advocated, in a revised Magnet model, the incorporation of **transformational leadership** (Wolf, Triolo, & Ponte, 2008). Defined by Burns (1978) as when "two or more persons engage with others in such a way that the leader and followers raise one another to high levels of motivation and morality" (p. 20), transformational leadership depends on a high level of engagement between the leader and followers.

Transformational leaders role model the following beliefs in their practice: **idealized influence**, which inspires high standards and outstanding professional practice, gaining the trust and respect of staff; **inspirational motivation**, which communicates a vision others wish to emulate; and **intellectual stimulation**, challenging staff to develop creative and innovative solutions and ways to provide growth and development opportunities. Additionally, transformational leaders are aware of individual staff members' career aspirations and are often in a position to guide individuals to invaluable mentoring opportunities (Heuston & Wolf, 2011; Luzinski, 2011).

In contrast, **transactional leadership** is based on an understanding between managers and employees regarding salary, benefits, and working conditions in exchange for job performance. The leader establishes goals, provides direction, and rewards employee progress in meeting goals by using praise and recognition, as well as merit increases and job promotion (McGuire & Kennerly, 2006). Leaders using a transactional style reward good behavior, punish perceived negative behavior, and maintain control at the top of the hierarchy.

Health care organizations have traditionally used transactional leadership strategies, which include a task-and-reward orientation, management by exception, few opportunities for creative thinking, decision making by senior management, and limited opportunities for employees to be involved. Although transactional leadership can help organizations meet their goals, evidence-based research (Weberg, 2010) supports transformational leadership, which can influence attitudes and behavior to create a new culture for nursing practice and patient care. Evidence demonstrates that groups led by transformational leaders have higher levels of performance and satisfaction than groups led by other types of leaders (Bass & Riggio, 2006).

QUALITIES OF THE TRANSFORMATIONAL LEADER

There are four components to transformational leadership, sometimes referred to as the 4 Is:

Idealized Influence (II): The leader serves as an ideal role model for followers; the leader "walks the talk" and is admired for this.

Inspirational Motivation (IM): Transformational leaders have the ability to inspire and motivate followers. Combining these first two Is is what constitutes the transformational leader's charisma.

Individualized Consideration (IC): Transformational leaders demonstrate genuine concern for the needs and feelings of followers. This personal attention to each follower is a key element in bringing out their very best efforts.

Intellectual Stimulation (IS): The leader challenges followers to be innovative and creative. A common misunderstanding is that transformational leaders are "soft," but the truth is that they constantly challenge followers to higher levels of performance.

Developing transformational leadership skills requires that nurse leaders be honest and reflective about their current practices. Dr. Ronald Riggio (Bass & Riggio, 2006), an expert in leadership development, encourages leaders to ask themselves the following to assess their transformational leader qualities: (Agree or Disagree).

Key: (Items 1 and 2 = II; 3 and 4 = IM; 5 and 6 = IC; 7 and 8 = IS)

1. I would never require a follower to do something that I wouldn't do myself.
2. My followers would say that they know what I stand for.
3. Inspiring others has always come easy to me.
4. My followers have told me that my enthusiasm and positive energy are infectious.
5. My followers would say that I am very attentive to their needs and concerns.
6. Even though I could easily do a task myself, I delegate it to expand my followers' skills.
7. Team creativity and innovation are the keys to success.
8. I encourage my followers to question their most basic ways of thinking.

Leadership is a journey of self-development, a work in progress. Transformational leaders focus on and care about followers, their personal needs, and their development. They possess high regard and expectations for staff and believe that they can do their best. In this way, transformational leaders inspire, empower, and stimulate followers to exceed levels of performance.

CHAPTER 7 REFLECTIVE QUESTIONS

1. What are the characteristics of the leaders whom you admire in your practice setting?

2. In considering the activities of the nurse managers in your practice setting, what management activities do they perform?

3. What are the experience and educational background of nurse managers at all levels of your organization? Do they have formal education in business or management?

4. How do the leaders in your work setting interact with each other and with the nursing staff?

5. What are the opportunities to become a leader within your own organization?

6. How could you best prepare for management responsibility?

7. How would you describe the differences between leader and manager roles?

8. In your opinion, which leadership theory is most appropriate for nursing practice? Why?

CHAPTER 8

Legal and Ethical Issues in Nursing

OBJECTIVES

1. Examine ethical principles in nursing.
2. Identify the Nurse Practice Act as the legal boundary of nursing.
3. Review the Code of Ethics for Nurses.
4. Describe the Patient Self-Determination Act (PSDA).
5. Explain the role of the nurse as client advocate.
6. Describe the process of informed consent.
7. Discuss the functions and sources of law as they relate to health care and professional nursing practice.
8. Contrast the differences between criminal and civil law.
9. Analyze the elements of malpractice and negligence and how they relate to nursing practice.
10. Consider strategies involved in preparing for and giving a deposition.

KEY TERMS

Accountability
Advocacy
Autonomy
Beneficence
Breach
Causation
Civil law
Client advocacy
Criminal law
Code of Ethics for Nurses
Damages

Delegation
Duty
Fidelity
Justice
Malpractice
Negligence
Situation/background/
    assessment/
    recommendation (SBAR)
Tort
Values clarification

STANDARDS

Patient-Centered Care		
Definition: Recognize the patient or designee as the source of control and full partner in providing compassionate and coordinated care based on respect for patient's preferences, values, and needs.		
Knowledge	**Skills**	**Attitudes**
Explore ethical and legal implications of patient-centered care. Describe the limits and boundaries of therapeutic patient-centered care	Recognize the boundaries of therapeutic relationships. Facilitate informed patient consent for care	Acknowledge the tension that may exist between patient rights and the organizational responsibility for professional, ethical care. Appreciate shared decision making with empowered patients and families, even when conflicts occur

This chapter presents a basic overview of the influence of law, legal issues, and the field of ethics and bioethics on the professional practice of nursing. With greater autonomy in practice settings, professional accountability and responsibility are of utmost concern in the nursing profession today. Consumers, too, are more knowledgeable and informed about their rights within the health care delivery system.

The information provided here is intended to highlight the impact of both ethics and law on the professional practice of nursing, the role of nursing in defining professional standards of care, and the legal guidelines that support nursing practice. Applying legal concepts within an ethical framework enhances client care through examining how these issues affect one's clinical practice.

BENEFICENCE AND FIDELITY

Recently a father arrived in our office to pick up his son's prescription. I noticed he appeared very upset, so I went out to the waiting room to bring him the script and to see if I could engage him in conversation. He proceeded to tell me that he was very worried about his son. I brought him into one of the exam rooms to discuss his concerns in a more private place. He expressed that his son was increasingly more depressed, getting into trouble, and avoiding family by staying out late with his friends or spending time alone in his room. Dad was concerned because he himself had a long history of depression. It took him years to feel comfortable enough to get help, and even longer to get the right dose of medication to work.

At this point Dad was teary-eyed and appeared very lost. Sitting next to him, occasionally nodding my head, I knew that I could not let this father leave in this state. I reassured him that addressing his concerns was the best decision. Although his primary care provider (PCP) was not currently in the building, the clinical support options (CSO) team was available. They gave Dad emergency mental health assistance information and advised that if he felt his son presented an immediate danger to himself or others, he should go to the nearest ED (emergency department) with him, or call 911. At this point, the father did not feel the situation was that dire. I scheduled his son for a follow-up with the PCP the next day as well as a referral to CSO. Dad left much less stressed.

Today the patient is currently in therapy and doing much better. It makes me happy to have been there to advocate for this family, and to have helped bring about such a positive outcome.

Nursing student

ETHICS IN NURSING

Treat people as if they were what they ought to be, and you help them to become what they are capable of being.

Johann Wolfgang von Goethe
Philosopher, poet, playwright

Ethics are the principles that guide an individual, group, or profession in conduct. **Bioethics** is a particular area of ethics concentrating on moral issues in the field of health care. **Nursing ethics** is sometimes viewed as a subgroup of bioethics because of the unique variety of ethical problems that arise in relation to working with clients, families, and other members of the health care team (Beauchamp & Childress, 2009).

Ethics deal with standards of conduct and moral judgment. The major principles of health care ethics that must be upheld in all situations are **autonomy, beneficence, nonmaleficence, justice,** and **fidelity.** Although nurses make independent decisions regarding client care, they are still responsible to the profession as a whole in how those decisions are made. Nightingale referred to specific issues of conduct and moral behavior. The Nightingale pledge (1860) includes the vow "to abstain from whatever is deleterious and mischievous and will not take or knowingly administer any harmful drug."

Autonomy is derived from the Latin meaning "auto" or "self," and "nomy" or "control." In the area of nursing, clients must be given the right to assist in their own decision making. It stands for independence and the ability to be self-directed. Clients have the right of self-determination and are entitled to decide what happens to them; therefore, competent adults have the capacity to consent to or refuse treatment. Nurses must respect the client's wishes, even if they may not agree with them.

In 1990, the Patient Self-Determination Act (PSDA) was passed by Congress (Walerius, Hill, & Anderson, 2009). This act stated that competent people could make their wishes known regarding the end-of-life experience. Also included in this act is the durable power of attorney, in which a competent person can assist in end-of-life decision making when the individual was no longer competent. In clinical situations, nurses respect the client's autonomy; here, the individual is given the freedom of choice regarding treatment. If a client is unable to make such a decision and has an advanced directive, the individual who has the durable power of attorney can make the decision.

Beneficence is the compassionate act of taking positive action to help others. As an essential principle of client advocacy, beneficence means to do good, not harm. Illustrated in the situation of an 18-year-old transported to the hospital following a bicycle accident, the emergency department (ED) nurse immediately administers prescribed pain medication in an act of beneficence. She obtains the consent for treatment while confirming that the client is cognizant of benefits and risks of any procedures that must be performed. She weighs the benefit of medicating the client for pain against obtaining a consent from a client that may not have the ability to make an informed decision for treatment.

Nonmaleficence is the concept of preventing intentional harm. In the American Nurses Association (ANA) Code for Nurses (2001), there is a specific duty to protect clients through reporting unsafe, illegal, or unethical practices. Nurses are often faced with making decisions about extending life with technology. Balancing potential client benefit with potential client harm is carried out in the decision-making process, as well as consideration of the client's wishes. The nurse must maintain a competent practice level to avoid causing injury or suffering to clients.

Additionally, the concept of nonmaleficence includes reporting suspected abuse to prevent further victimization. As the core of medical oath and nursing ethics, nonmaleficence encompasses avoidance of harm.

The ethical principle of **justice** compels health care providers to treat clients equally and fairly. Nurses are continually confronted with matters of justice when planning and delivering client care, considering the amount of time to be spent with each based on client needs and nursing resources. This principle refers to an equal and fair distribution of resources, based on analysis of benefits and burdens of decision. Justice indicates that all clients have an equal right to the services delivered, regardless of client status or contributions.

Based upon the virtue of caring, **fidelity** involves an agreement to keep a promise. This principle requires loyalty, fairness, truthfulness, advocacy, and dedication to our patients (Beauchamp & Childress, 2009). Privacy and confidentiality are concepts that could be challenged under the concept of fidelity. If a nurse is aware of another health care provider who is impaired, but the circumstances are private or confidential, how is the conflict resolved?

Nurses need to distinguish between their personal values and their professional ethics. Personal values are what nurses hold significant and true for themselves, while professional ethics involve principles that have universal applications and standards of conduct that must be upheld in all situations. Nurses thus avoid allowing personal judgments to bias client care. They are honest and fair with clients, and they act in the best interests of and show respect for clients.

Developed in 1985, the Code of Ethics for Nurses outlines responsibilities and conduct expected of practicing nurses. Nurses are responsible for complying with the standards of ethical practice; as well, they safeguard other nurses' compliance with these standards. Code revisions in 2001 incorporated advancing nursing science matters, based on the input of nurses practicing in a variety of settings. The ANA (2001) endorsed nine terms that concentrate on ethical practice issues: compassion and respect; commitment to the client; client advocacy, responsibility, and accountability; duties; participation in the health care setting; advancement of the profession; and collaboration.

CLIENT ADVOCACY

All of the issues and responsibilities that encompass the nursing role can be summarized in the words "client advocate." Nurses are the primary system support for their clients, from initial admission to eventual discharge. In easing the client's transition from treatment in the ED, through admission to the unit, to providing consistent emotional support, nurses are on the front line, advocating for clients.

Client advocacy includes a therapeutic relationship and communication between nurse and client and can involve acting on behalf of a client. The nurse's role as liaison bridges the communication gap with the client, other professions, and the health care system. However, nurses may find that advocating for clients is sometimes challenged by administration, physicians, and nursing peers. Some nurses see the consequences of nursing advocacy as risk taking. To overcome this obstacle, nurses are encouraged to use clear, effective communication when advocating for clients. Statements will be better received when points are clearly articulated (Mahlin, 2010).

During the hospital experience, communication and education become most important. Clients need to understand the tests and procedures being ordered, how long these tests will take, and why the tests are being done in the first place. As client advocates, nurses interpret for clients in terms they can understand. "NPO r/t N/V and 4 mg Zofran" can be frightening to the client until the nurse translates, "You will have nothing to eat or drink right now related to your nausea and vomiting, and you will be given some medication to relieve your nausea."

All health care providers have an ethical duty to support and empower their clients; it is an expected competency for practicing nurses. Through incorporating therapeutic communication skills, building a strong foundation of resources for clients, families, and health care providers, and following ethical principles in their daily practices, nurses can truly become effective client advocates.

LEGAL ISSUES IN NURSING

Nurses need to understand how the legal system works to be safe and effective providers of care. The professions of law and nursing are both committed to helping clients and society. The collaboration of law and nursing is necessary for achieving effective outcomes for both the nurse and the client.

Nurse practice acts control the practice of nursing through licensure. They legally define the practice of nursing within each state, describing the scope of nursing practice and protecting the public. Accountability is an essential concept of professional practice under the law. Nurses need to understand laws that regulate and affect practice to ensure that their actions are consistent with current legal principles and to protect themselves from liability.

Competence in nursing practice is determined and maintained by various credentialing methods, including licensure, registration, certification, and accreditation. The purpose of these credentialing methods is to protect the public's welfare and safety.

Three of the most common areas of the law that may affect nurses include **civil law, criminal law,** and **agency law.**

Civil law describes the private rights and responsibilities of individuals. The "plaintiff" initiates the lawsuit against the "defendant." Civil lawsuits may involve actions in contracts, property, and torts. **Torts** concern a private or civil wrong that causes injury as a result of disregard for a duty an individual had to another person. Tort lawsuits usually involve personal injuries and, while not criminal, may involve actions similar to criminal acts, punishable in a separate legal action. In civil law, the defendant may be found liable and forced to pay the plaintiff for the damages caused. Nursing malpractice and employment actions involve civil laws.

Criminal law involves crimes and punishments. The state or federal government brings a charge against a defendant, who if found guilty may be required to pay a fine to the government and/or complete a prison sentence. Unlike the monetary settlement in a civil lawsuit, the outcome of criminal law is punishment.

Originating from the government's legislative branch, **agency law** cases usually involve the monitoring and managing of certain areas of regulation, such as the state board of nursing. Clients may bring complaints regarding nursing care to the state board, which may discipline nurses. In this instance, the client does not receive monetary compensation.

NEGLIGENCE AND MALPRACTICE

The Joint Commission (TJC) defines negligence as "failure to use such care as a reasonably prudent and careful person would use under similar circumstances" and malpractice as "improper or unethical conduct or unreasonable lack of skill by a holder of a professional or official position; often applied to physicians, dentists, lawyers, and public officers to denote negligent or unskillful performance of duties when professional skills are obligatory." The Commission's definition further states: "Malpractice is a cause of action for which damages are allowed" (Stubenrauch, 2007, p. 63).

Most lawsuits against nurses are for alleged violations of tort law. In general terms, a tort is an action or omission that harms someone. According to Helm (2003), a tort is a civil wrong or injury resulting from a breach of legal duty that exists by virtue of society's expectations regarding interpersonal conduct or by the assumption of a duty inherent in a professional relationship (as opposed to a legal duty that exists by virtue of a contractual relationship). Malpractice refers to a tort committed by a professional acting in his or her professional capacity. The law distinguishes between unintentional and intentional torts. An unintentional tort results from negligence. In contrast, "an intentional tort is a deliberate invasion of someone's legal right. In a malpractice case involving an intentional tort, the plaintiff doesn't need to prove that you owed him a duty. [The duty] is defined by law, and you are presumed to owe him this duty." In such a case, the plaintiff has to show only that the defendant breached his or her duty and that the breach caused the plaintiff harm. Examples of intentional torts include assault, battery, false imprisonment, invasion of privacy, and slander.

Negligence is either an act of omission (not doing something a reasonably prudent person would do) or commission (doing something a reasonably prudent person would not do). Malpractice is negligence by a professional. Four elements are needed to prove malpractice:

1. **Duty**: Duty stands for a legal obligation owed by one person to another person. When nurses care for clients, they assume the duty to care for them in a competent and diligent manner. Nurses are expected to provide the degree of care ordinarily exercised by other nurses practicing in the same nursing specialty. Therefore, nurses are expected to adhere to standards of care—those imposed by the nurse's state board of nursing nurse practice act; the national nursing specialty standards of care and scope of practice; and the nurse's hospital, or other agency, protocols.

2. **Breach**: A breach of duty takes place when there is failure to fulfill the duties established as being the responsibility of the nurse. In other words, nurses breach their duty when they do not meet the appropriate standard of care.

3. **Causation**: Causation is the most difficult element to prove because it is the factual connection between what the nurse did and the injury to the client. Causation means that the nurse's breach of duty, or failure to meet the appropriate standard of care, caused the client's injury or adverse outcome.

4. **Damages**: Damages are monetary payments designed to compensate the client for the injury or adverse outcome, and are intended to restore the plaintiff to his or her condition prior to the injury. To recover damages, the client must establish that he or she suffered physical, financial, or emotional injury caused by the nurse's violation of the standard of care. Damages are usually compensatory or punitive.

Croke (2003) has identified six major categories of negligence resulting in malpractice.

1. **Failure to follow standards of care**: Failure to perform a complete admission assessment or design a plan of care; adhere to standardized protocols or institutional policies and procedures; or follow a physician's verbal or written orders.

2. **Failure to use equipment in a responsible manner:** Failure to follow the manufacturer's recommendations for operating equipment; check equipment for safety prior to use; place equipment properly during treatment; or learn how equipment functions.

3. **Failure to communicate**: Failure to notify a physician in a timely manner when conditions warrant it; listen to a client's complaints and act on them; communicate effectively with a client; or seek higher medical authorization for a treatment.

4. **Failure to document**: Failure to note in the patient's medical record a client's progress and response to treatment; client's injuries; pertinent nursing assessment information; physician's medical orders; or information on telephone conversations with physicians, including time, content of communication between nurse and physician, and actions taken.

5. **Failure to assess and monitor**: Failure to complete a shift assessment; implement a plan of care; observe a client's ongoing progress; or interpret a client's signs and symptoms.

6. **Failure to act as a patient advocate:** Failure to question discharge orders when a client's condition warrants it; question incomplete or illegible medical orders; or provide a safe environment.

PRINCIPLES FOR LEGAL PROTECTION IN NURSING PRACTICE

Legal actions against nurses can occur when a client claims that the nurse breached a standard of care, which can result in harm to the client. Observing the following practices can protect the nurse legally (Austin, 2008).

Medication errors compromise the safety of clients and can result in extended hospital stays, lawsuits, and compensation for damages. An awareness on the part of the nurse of the medication given is a basic element in the nursing standard of practice for medication therapy. Agencies can employ procedures such as independent double checks to help prevent errors associated with single-unit doses of high-alert medications. An example of this may involve one nurse drawing up the medication while another nurse verifies that the medication, dose, and route are correct. Both nurses document the entry in the electronic medication administration record (MAR).

Changes in the client's condition indicate the need for timely assessment, monitoring, reporting, and documentation. Vigilance is a state of watchful attention. This ability to detect danger leads to a readiness to act (Meyer & Lavin, 2005). Vigilance includes attention to and identification of clinically significant observations/signals/cues; calculation of risk inherent in nursing practice situations; and the readiness to act appropriately and efficiently to minimize risks and to respond to threats.

Nightingale (1860) cited the importance of vigilance in nursing: "The most important practical lesson that can be given to nurses is to teach them what to observe—how to observe—what symptoms indicate improvement—what the reverse—which are of importance—which are of none—which are evidence of neglect—and of what kind of neglect. All this is what ought to make part, and an essential part, of the training of every nurse" (*Notes on Nursing*, p. 105).

Ignoring worsening signs and symptoms in a client can result in legal actions brought against nurses. The inability to recognize and communicate the significance of the client's deteriorating condition is considered failure to rescue (Clarke & Aiken, 2003). To rescue a patient appropriately, the nurse "must be able to anticipate when complications are likely to occur and rapidly recognize cues that indicate that problems are beginning" (p.43).

Effective communication is key when "handing off" client care to another nurse, speaking with a client, and interacting with a client's family. In working with a client who has limited proficiency in English, the nurse relies on the hospital's medical interpreter to translate instructions to the client. If a competent medical language interpreter is not provided, the nurse could face charges of substandard nursing care.

TJC (Dayton & Henriksen, 2007) has set a standard for communication when one caregiver transfers patient care to another caregiver. According to their requirements, the nurse transferring care must give the nurse taking responsibility for the patient all appropriate information about the patient's condition, response to treatment during the shift, changes in condition or treatment plan, and any other information that will help the next nurse plan for the patient's care.

SBAR: SITUATION, BACKGROUND, ASSESSMENT, RECOMMENDATION

To ensure an efficient and comprehensive client report, the **SBAR** method is recommended: **situation** (identify the client and why admitted); **background** (concise history, tests/treatments completed); **assessment** (client's current status); **recommendation** (client's plan of care).

When **delegating responsibly,** the nurse must be aware of team members' appropriate skills and competencies to meet the needs of the client when assigning care. When creating the daily assignment, the nurse must delegate appropriately and supervise the person carrying out the assignment. To delegate safely, nurses must also understand what the state board of nursing allows in assigning other members of the health care team to client care. The five rights for delegating to another caregiver provide an easy-to-remember guide: right person, right task, right circumstances, right direction, and right supervision. The nurse may need to intervene in the care being given. The nurse must remain responsible for clients and evaluate condition and response to the tasks performed.

Precise, timely documentation in the client's medical record is critical. It is a legal document required by state laws and regulations. The record provides a means of communication among caregivers that ensures continuity of care. Additionally, it is used for education and research and to substantiate insurance reimbursement claims, and can be used as evidence in legal proceedings to establish whether or not the care rendered met the legal standard of care.

A basic rule of safe documentation is to know and follow the agency's documentation policies and procedures. Failure to follow facility policy can result in inconsistencies, may compromise patient safety, and may create legal problems if the record ends up in court. Regardless of how professional a nurse appears on the witness stand, careless documentation can make a profoundly negative impression on a jury.

Following institutional policies and procedures helps establish the nursing standards of care held to in court. Client care policies and procedures must be based on current and recognized practice. They must be updated regularly, and they should be realistic. Any deviation from a policy or procedure that harms the client can subject you and the facility to liability exposure, so some flexibility is necessary. As well, nurses have an obligation to ensure they have received orientation and education on all equipment used to provide client care: intended use, proper operation, and policies and procedures for using it if they exist.

PREPARING FOR A DEPOSITION

Nurses are often summoned as deposition witnesses. Identified as a party in a lawsuit, staff member in a defendant hospital, or as an expert, testimony by nurses typically involves civil cases in personal injury, medical malpractice, and nursing negligence. Criminal cases include elder abuse, sexual assault, and domestic violence.

As expert witnesses and legal nurse consultants, nurses' testimonies involve clinical practice and standards of care. The American Bar Association reports that over 95% of cases are settled prior to trial (Barkai & Martin, 2006). Deposition, a sworn testimony that conveys the same effect if given before a judge and jury, can be carried out in a home, hospital, or law office. Nurses provide testimony that can be crucial to either the defense or plaintiff in a medical malpractice case. The testimony validates and amplifies the facts in the medical record.

To prepare for the deposition, the nurse should review the chart and any other information recommended by legal counsel. Hospital lawyers represent the organization and, occasionally, the nurse as agent for the hospital. However, if the deposition concerns nursing negligence, the nurse may be named party in the lawsuit. If not provided, the nurse should consider hiring a lawyer for the deposition (Reising & Allen, 2007).

The testimony itself is executed in a question-and-answer format. The nurse should listen to the complete question posed by the examining lawyer before responding, and answer only the question asked. If the question calls for an explanation, it is appropriate to give one. A judge or jury will be listening/reading/watching the nurse's deposition. A nurse who believes a clinical detail is important for the legal record should notify his or her lawyer. If central to the case, the nurse's attorney will ask questions related to the clinical detail after the examining lawyer has finished his or her portion of the deposition.

It is acceptable for the nurse to give his or her "best recollection" (Brooke, 2006, p. 46). However, the nurse must clarify for the record that he or she is giving a best estimate of what occurred. Staying focused and remaining calm are crucial elements during examination testimony. The nurse may request breaks if needed to avoid undue stress and exhaustion, which could compromise accuracy and, ultimately, the outcome of the deposition.

At the conclusion of the questions by the examining lawyer, the other lawyers in the case will have an opportunity to ask the nurse questions. Once everyone has exhausted their list of questions, the nurse will "go off the record" and the deposition will end. The court reporter transcribes the deposition into booklet form; a copy is made available for the nurse's review and comment.

Knowing what to expect at a deposition and being aware of some of the most common concerns and issues can eliminate much of the mystery and fear for nurses. Familiarity with the process will help ensure an accurate testimony reflective of the situation in question.

CHAPTER 8 REFLECTIVE QUESTIONS

1. Describe an ethical legal situation that you have experienced in your life. How did this make you feel? If you were to experience this again, is there anything you would do differently? Why/why not?

2. Review the Code of Ethics for Nurses with Interpretive Statements (http://www.nursingworld.org/codeofethics). How do you incorporate this document in daily nursing practice? Would you add any conditions to the document? Why/why not?

3. Give examples of how the major principles of health care ethics (autonomy, beneficence, nonmaleficence, justice, and fidelity) are incorporated into your daily nursing practice.

4. What has been your experience with the acronym SBAR? If SBAR is new to you, would you consider implementing it in your workplace setting? Give reasons for your answer.

5. Malpractice is negligence by a professional, but not all malpractice is negligence (Stubenrauch, 2007). Construct a legal situation in nursing, incorporating examples of the four elements (duty, breach, causation, and damages) needed to prove malpractice.

PART IV

Skill Competencies for the Baccalaureate-Prepared Nurse

CHAPTER 9

Information Technology in Nursing

OBJECTIVES

1. Define nursing informatics and technology assessment.
2. Identify applications of information technology and health care.
3. Discuss the Technology Informatics Guiding Education Reform (TIGER) Movement.
4. Analyze current trends in nursing education designed to integrate informatics into the nursing curriculum.

KEY TERMS

Debriefing

Discussion board

Electronic health record (EHR)

Hospital information system (HIS)

Netiquette

Nursing Informatics Education Model (NIEM)

PowerPoint presentations

Simulated E-Health Delivery System (SEEDS)

Simulation

Technology Informatics Guiding Educational Reform (TIGER)

STANDARDS

Informatics		
Definition: Use information and technology to communicate, manage knowledge, mitigate error, and support decision making.		
Knowledge	Skills	Attitudes
Explain why information and technology skills are essential for safe patient care	Seek education about how information is managed in care settings before providing care. Apply technology and information management tools to support safe processes of care	Appreciate the necessity for all health professionals to seek lifelong, continuous learning of information technology skills
Identify essential information that must be available in a common database to support patient care. Contrast benefits and limitations of different communication technologies and their impact on safety and quality	Navigate the electronic health record. Document and plan patient care in an electronic health record Employ communication technologies to coordinate care for patients	Value technologies that support clinical decision making, error prevention, and care coordination. Protect confidentiality of protected health information in electronic health records
Describe examples of how technology and information management is related to the quality and safety of patient care. Recognize the time, effort, and skill required for computers, databases, and other technologies to become reliable and effective tools for patient care	Respond appropriately to clinical decision-making supports and alerts. Use information management tools to monitor outcomes of care processes Use high-quality electronic sources of health care information	Value nurses' involvement in design, selection, implementation, and evaluation of information technologies to support patient care

Technology is nothing. What's important is that you have a faith in people, that they're basically good and smart, and if you give them tools, they'll do wonderful things with them.

Steve Jobs

TECHNOLOGY GROWING PAINS

I can sympathize with the workloads that we all encounter; however, it is imperative that we document accurately for the safety of our patients and the integrity of our license. Currently I am working with the nursing informatics team at my hospital to develop an EMR. One of our main objectives is to find "meaningful use" in the assessments, interventions, and orders we build. How can we ensure that what we document is being relayed to the next shift or the other disciplines caring for the patient? As we try to streamline our documentation and make things uniform as to avoid duplicate information, many times it is difficult to communicate subtle changes in patient status.

Nursing student

This chapter provides an introduction to nursing informatics (NI), the organization of data, information, and knowledge important to nursing (American Nurses Association [ANA], 2008b). The content here examines the responsibilities, challenges, and opportunities presented to the nurse in working with information systems at the point of care; the importance of attending educational programs to expand knowledge on and to impact nursing practice; and the management of continuously evolving research data.

Technology is here and here to stay. Nurses must embrace and integrate technology skills into their daily professional practice. Informatics technology strengthens an evidence-based approach through open, complete, and current access to continuously emerging data surrounding the nursing profession. The ability of nurses to use and to manage information systems is crucial to improving outcomes, decreasing costs, and improving access to care (Institute of Medicine [IOM], 2001).

THE GROWTH OF INFORMATICS COMPETENCIES IN NURSING

With the incorporation of electronic health records (EHRs) into health care professions, nursing is challenged to build informatics competencies into their knowledge base (Hart, 2010). Given the present clinical climate, this necessitates considerable review and redesign of nursing curricula in order for both students and faculty to remain current in an environment of rapidly changing technology. Informatics technology (IT) is no longer a recommended addition to current nursing curricula; it must be integrated into all clinical courses. Where to place this information, and what material to eliminate to make room for an IT education module, present a daunting challenge, however. Nursing faculty are charged with the responsibility of incorporating informatics skills into an already overburdened curriculum (Vestal, Krautwurst, & Hack, 2008; Warfield, 2008). Nonetheless, giving nursing students the information regarding how to practice in an informatics, evidence-based, client-centered health care environment is vital.

Frequently students and instructors are introduced to the informatics model in the clinical setting without the time and resources needed to adequately orient to the system, and without the information systems department personnel to provide secure access to the system (Melo & Carlton, 2008). Valuable time and energy is spent trouble-shooting computer problems while on the job, which takes nursing students away from the hands-on practice and refinement of nursing skills needed to complete the objectives for the clinical component of the course. It involves the time and patience of nursing staff on the clinical unit to repair the computer problems caused by well-intentioned novices. The outcomes of an integrated technology curriculum provide the chance to positively impact nursing education and to provide graduates with the competencies and leadership for improving quality and safety in patient care (Smedley, 2005).

The need to integrate nursing and IT is not a new initiative. Calling for a major change in health care practices, the IOM published *To Err is Human* in the year 2000 (IOM, 2000). This report became the incentive in a series of publications on client safety, quality, efficiency, and the use of information technologies. In 2003, a second IOM report, *Health Professional Education: A Bridge to Quality*, cited the need for major changes in health care education. The authors advised that without a concentration in informatics competencies, health care professionals would be extremely limited to make competent use of communication and information technology skills (IOM, 2003).

In response to this challenge, a jointly funded partnership entitled *SEEDS: Simulated E-Health Delivery System* (Warren & Connors, 2007) formed between the school of nursing at the University of Kansas and the Cerner Corporation, a health care information technology supplier. Addressing both teaching and learning strategies in education and technology, the partnership program provided tools to help nursing students obtain information technology skills, thereby enhancing their clinical experience. Program director Judith J. Warren, PhD, RN, modified EHR software to foster student learning in relation to informatics skills and client information management. Faculty participation involved such learning activities as assessment, documentation of skills, care planning, and drug information management for integration in the SEEDS program. From this initiative, three other nursing schools implemented the program. This group went on to establish the Academic Education Solution Consortium (AESC), with the goal of creating a link between classroom and clinical experiences in nursing education (Warren & Connors, 2007).

Saba and Riley (Saba & Riley, 1997; Saba & McCormick, 2006) created the Nursing Informatics Education Model (NIEM), in which computer, information, and nursing sciences are woven throughout the curriculum to ensure the development of NI technologies. Nursing students are able to learn, practice, and refine skills related to computer literacy in their initial coursework. In subsequent coursework, students advance to the intricacies of information management and their connection to the clinical environment.

Additional agencies have made significant contributions to the challenge. Following the IOM report, the National League for Nursing (NLN) established the Task Group on Informatics Competencies (NLN, 2008). When conducting a literature search on informatics competencies for the different levels of education, the task force discovered that while competencies were identified, nursing schools demonstrated "limited adoption" of the competencies. A survey to determine the extent to which current nursing curricula prepare students with informatics competencies revealed that while most schools of nursing focused on computer and information literacy, there was limited involvement in the attainment of informatics knowledge and skills.

In their report, *Preparing the Next Generation of Nurses to Practice in a Technology-Rich Environment: An Informatics Agenda* (NLN, 2008), the NLN includes the following recommendations for nursing faculty: (a) participate in faculty development programs to achieve competency in informatics; (b) incorporate informatics into the curriculum; (c) achieve competency through participation in faculty development programs; (d) partner with clinicians and informatics people at clinical agencies to help faculty and students; (e) collaborate with clinical agencies to ensure that students have hands-on experience with informatics tools; and (f) collaborate with clinical agencies to demonstrate transformations in clinical practice produced by informatics.

The Quality and Safety Education for Nurses (QSEN) program was created in 2005 by an expert panel of nursing educators with the aim of preparing future nurses to continuously advance the quality and safety of the health care system in which they practice (Cronenwett & Sherwood, 2007). The group developed six core competencies to be incorporated into nursing curricula: client-centered care; teamwork and collaboration; evidence-based practice; quality improvement; safety; and informatics.

In the first phase of the QSEN initiative, educators sought national consensus on definitions of quality and safety competencies to institute changes in nursing education for all registered nurses. In the second phase, the panel surveyed schools of nursing to determine which of the six core competencies are already included in curricula, whether faculty are equipped to teach these competencies, and how well nursing students are learning them. The third phase of the QSEN project involves developing faculty expertise to teach the competencies; placing the six competencies in textbooks, licensing, accreditation, and certification standards; and endorsing sustained innovation in teaching the six core competencies.

THE TECHNOLOGY INFORMATICS GUIDING EDUCATION REFORM (TIGER) MOVEMENT

The Office of the National Coordinator of Health Information Technology was established in 2004 to continue to advance the agenda of integrating IT into nursing curricula; however, even though nursing had for years provided continuous support for the field of NI, the profession was ignored when the plan was released. This exclusion moved several nursing leaders to create the Technology Informatics Guiding Education Reform (TIGER) movement. In 2006, the TIGER initiative began as a grassroots effort in response not only to the rebuff from the Office of the National Coordinator of Health Information Technology, but as a reaction to President Bush's 2004 challenge to the U.S. health care industry to establish electronic medical records for everyone by the year 2014.

Over 100 leaders from nursing administration, practice, education, informatics, technology organizations, and government agencies met to create a vision for the future of nursing. Their objective involved pairing information technology and health care professions to address the challenge of providing safer, more effective, quality patient care. Participants identified seven critical factors for achieving this vision: leadership that drives the transformation of health care; collaborative learning communities that maximize knowledge development and dissemination; standardized, person-centered, technology-enabled processes fostering teamwork across the continuum of care; evidence-based, interoperable intelligence systems supporting education and practice; people-centered, affordable universal technologies; consistent, incentives-based initiatives supporting coalition building; and an open system covering technology and informatics across multiple disciplines (TIGER, 2008).

Members of this initiative have worked tirelessly to support implementation of informatics competencies for all levels of nursing education and practice. The TIGER organization strives to ensure that all nurses and nursing students are educated in using informatics, education that will return nurses to the bedside in the delivery of safer, higher-quality patient care. More nursing care means fewer complications, lower mortality rates, and shorter hospital stays, with the potential to prevent over 6,700 patient deaths and four million hospital days a year (TIGER, 2008).

As the health care industry moves toward adopting electronic medical records, the nursing profession must ensure that informatics competencies are part of every nurse's skill set. It will require that all nursing organizations work together to make this happen, to incorporate informatics into nursing, and to make IT the "stethoscope" of the 21st century (TIGER, 2008).

As the IOM stressed in its reports, utilizing informatics is a core competency required of all health care professions. These competencies must be incorporated into education at every level and into daily practice, requiring partnership and commitment across nursing: "It is high time to embrace a collaborative approach to educational reform. The profession and, most importantly, the patient will be the beneficiaries" (IOM, 2003).

INTEGRATING INFORMATION TECHNOLOGY IN EDUCATION AND PRACTICE

Nursing is continually experiencing evolution and transformation. As health care changes, the way nursing students and novice nurses are educated must change as well. These adaptations are necessary to meet the needs of the health care client and to provide quality care. Technology is a significant factor in health care and education. Although the literature proliferates regarding recommendations and guidelines in technology integration, the actual education surrounding the process has yet to match this growth (Nguyen, Zierler, & Nguyen, 2011).

Informatics is considered a core competency for nursing and allied health program educators by both the IOM (2010) and the NLN (2008). Effective health care requires timely information to allow for critical thinking and decision making on the part of the new nurse. With the growth of technology, it is vital for faculty to effectively engage today's contemporary learners in the classroom. Nursing faculty members are challenged to develop and educate professionals who are ready to effectively use mobile technology to ascertain the information they need to provide quality care.

INTEGRATING INFORMATICS INTO THE NURSING CURRICULUM

Simulation Education

Even in the most cooperative of learning environments in nursing academia, it seems that content is delivered in fragments. In class and clinical settings (if time and experiences present themselves), students learn about hemorrhage, fluid loss, IV replacement fluids, indications for catheterization, use of oxygen, and so on; but when it comes time to prioritize, to put the pieces together, and to professionally react to an emergency situation, often students do not know where to begin.

The following narrative highlights the benefits of a simulation scenario in fostering the development of professionalism in nursing students. Professionalism embraces a set of attitudes, skills and behaviors, attributes, and values expected from those to whom society considers experts. The core values of professionalism include honesty and integrity, altruism, respect, responsibility and accountability, compassion and empathy, dedication, and self-improvement (Hendelman, 2009). Research has shown that simulation-based training can improve student learning, and therefore patient care (Cant & Cooper, 2010; Hodge, Martin, Tavernier, Perea-Ryan, & Van Houten, 2008; NLN, 2010, 2011). With the outcomes of improved student learning and better patient care, can simulation foster professionalism as well?

Faculty in nursing education are charged with the daunting task of equipping students with the skills to think critically, and to advance to synthesis and application of knowledge as they use the nursing process to deliver professional, responsible, individualized nursing care

(King, Hindenlang, Moseley, & Kuritz, 2008). Simulation provides a valuable addition to the traditional teacher-centered approach to nursing education (Cant & Cooper, 2010).

Through the expert assistance of a skilled, supportive nursing laboratory coordinator, nursing faculty members at one university have incorporated simulation as part of both clinical and classroom responsibilities in teaching the Maternal and Newborn course. Such a scenario takes place during the last 2 weeks of the semester, when postpartum complications are discussed. One such complication involves the hospitalized new mother experiencing a postpartum hemorrhage. Students are given a preliminary introduction to the scenario the day before the session. Roles are assigned the day of the scenario, to include primary nurse, secondary nurse, night nurse, nursing supervisor, and visitor. Audience members view the scenario from a separate room where the scenario is "streamed." Such a scenario accommodates up to eight students at one time. Before the 20- to 30-minute session starts, those who are in the scene itself are given the opportunity to enter the actual physical environment to orient and familiarize themselves with the setting.

Debriefing immediately after the scenario helps to clarify, amplify, and highlight each component of the simulation educational experience. Feedback corrects any misinformation or improper practice techniques. Gaps in knowledge are identified in individual students that would otherwise go undetected. With debriefing after the scenario, students feel that their opinions matter (Neill & Wotton, 2011). Each time the scenario is carried out, improvements are made based on debriefing sessions, meetings with nursing colleagues, video streaming of the event, and documenting students' evaluations of the scenario to generate the data needed to support the use of this teaching methodology. Students' "takeaways" from the experience include: surprise that faculty value student feedback and the importance of team, communication, and patient advocacy. These are all key to professionalism in practice.

In the "debriefing" after the scenario, professional growth was identified and articulated by the **students** themselves in the following areas:

Assessment skills: "Recognition early on of a developing problem"

Nursing skills (not an exhaustive list): "Communication, vital signs, medications, IV fluids, catheterization, oxygen administration"

Prioritizing: "I started to panic . . . what needs to be done first?"

Role playing (from a student audience member): "I was so impressed by the other students' actions . . . stepping up to the plate . . . getting right into the situation . . . I don't know if I would be able to step into their shoes as well if it were me in the 'hot seat.'"

Importance of team: "We needed each other for support . . . we needed help to safely care for this patient."

Delegation and management of resources: Recognizing that "one person cannot do it all"

Communication: With patient, nurse, supervisor, doctor, family . . . "Do you think we will ever get to this skill level?"

Decision making: "She (student as primary nurse) seemed so calm through it all!"

Ethics/patient advocacy (beneficence, fidelity, justice, respect for the patient and family members/visitors present): "I noticed how the secondary kept the patient informed each step of the way."

Conflict resolution: Dealing with members of the health care team, patients, and family members: "As the supervisor, he was very convincing in the role . . . he very professionally and confidently explained to the visitor the reason she had to leave."

Faculty in nursing education are charged with the daunting task of equipping students with the skills to think critically and to apply knowledge as they use the nursing process to deliver professional, responsible, individualized nursing care. Simulation provides a valuable addition to the traditional teacher-centered approach to nursing education. The emphasis is placed on the learning needs and preferences of current students, the majority of whom have been raised with technology (Nguyen et al., 2011).

Simulation helps nursing students to see the "big picture." The SIMS experience brings students closer to the attainment of professional skills, which in turn brings them closer to understanding the professional role of the registered nurse. Where better to practice and refine skills than in a controlled, safe setting where students can examine and improve on their practice?

Moreover, simulation scenarios permit faculty to involve students in situations that they may never witness in the clinical setting. Because students are placed in a variety of units for their clinical experiences, there is a lack of consistency in learning opportunities across and among students. The use of structured simulation scenarios affords nursing educators a unique opportunity to provide students with consistency in their learning experiences (Hodge et al., 2008).

Implications for future research include the following:

- "Success stories": Encourage faculty to publish/present their incorporation of simulation education into the curriculum
- Allot more time into the curriculum for simulation education
- Allocation of resources to assist overburdened simulation laboratory staff (typically one individual is responsible for maintaining the lab, scheduling teaching sessions, providing open labs, giving tours during open lab, ordering materials, and organizing remediation)
- Provide nursing faculty the opportunity and funding to attend conferences related to integrating simulation education into the curriculum, along with the benefits of "buying into" this adjunct to traditional nursing education
- More research studies on the many benefits of simulation education
- The involvement of students in creating scenarios/case studies as part of their integration of technology into the curriculum

Professionalism can be taught in the curriculum by encouraging and allowing faculty and students to have conversations about real-life events that challenge ideas of what it means to be a nurse. Challenges for students today include making the transition from passive to active learners, recognizing events that reflect professional behavior, talking with others about them, and becoming their own teachers of professionalism (Billings & Halstead, 2011; IOM, 2010).

Creating an Effective PowerPoint Presentation

To communicate a message or a story, PowerPoint presentations break the information down into snapshots. Each is a blank canvas for the pictures, words, and shapes that will help you build your story. Plan your PowerPoint presentation carefully by researching ahead of time, knowing your audience, and practicing your presentation before delivering it.

As you begin preparing a PowerPoint presentation, consider your audience. Adapt your message according to the current knowledge level the audience possesses on the topic. Focus on letting your words do the explaining, especially when it comes to persuading them on any complex ideas you need to convey. For the audience to understand the presentation intellectually as well as emotionally, the information must be conveyed to them as a well-organized, meaningful story.

Slide Total. To maintain a clear message and to keep your audience attentive and interested, keep the number of slides in your presentation to a minimum. You will lose your audience with too many slides. Include only necessary information. When introducing each new slide, afford the audience time to process the information on that slide. When an audience stops paying attention, the presentation loses its effectiveness. The ideal PowerPoint presentation should last no longer than 20 minutes (Kawasaki, 2012). Allow time for a question-and-answer period following the presentation.

Color. Look for ways color combinations can assist you in delivering both the contextual detail and the emotional impact in each slide you craft, so they support your message succinctly, clearly, and intuitively. A vivid contrast or a soothing balance might be called for to help make your points. Check all colors on a projection screen before giving the actual presentation. The colors may project differently than what appears on your monitor.

Font. Choose a font style that audience members can read from a distance. Choosing the right font style helps to best convey your message. Larger font indicates more important information. Kawasaki (2012) recommends a font size no smaller than 30 point. This size not only enhances visual clarity but prevents a tendency to add too much information on an individual slide.

Text. Keep text simple by using bulleted points or short sentences, keeping each to one line. It is recommended that no more than 6 bulleted points should be placed on each slide. Your audience should be listening to your presentation, not reading the screen. Some projectors crop slides at the edges, so long sentences may be cropped. Remove articles such as "a" and "the" to help reduce word count on a line. To earn and maintain the respect of your audience, always check the spelling and grammar in your presentation.

Graphics. Graphics help tell the story by enhancing and complementing the text. Overdoing graphics can overwhelm the slide and the audience. Do not use more than two graphics per slide. Label charts and graphs with enough text to make elements comprehensible. Slide backgrounds should be subtle and consistent. Use high contrast between background and text colors.

Delivering an Effective PowerPoint Presentation

Arrive Early. Verify that everything for your PowerPoint presentation works properly. Ensure that all equipment is connected and running. Do not assume that your presentation will work fine on another computer.

Technology Support. Establish with conference organizers if there will be available technology support before or during your presentation. If the computer with which you plan to give your presentation does not belong to you, make sure you understand how the equipment works.

Audience. Keep the audience focused on the content of your presentation. Monitor your audience's behavior. If audience members seem to be focusing only on the slides, they may be overwhelmed, confused, or distracted by too much slide content.

Questions. Before beginning the actual presentation, ask audience members to hold questions until the end. Questions are an excellent indicator that people are engaged by your subject matter and presentation skills. Holding questions until the end of the presentation increases the likelihood that you will get through your material uninterrupted.

Presentation Skills. Do not read your presentation. This action conveys a message of insecurity, disinterest, or unpreparedness on the speaker's part. Practice the presentation so that you can speak from the bulleted points. The text should be a guide for the presenter rather than the full message for the audience.

Timing. Stay on point. If you plan a certain amount of time for your presentation, do not go over. If there is no time limit, take less time rather than more to ensure that people stay engaged. Reserve enough time in the presentation for a question-and-answer period.

Inspiration. Motivate your audience by giving them an emotional connection to the information being presented. Showing enthusiasm demonstrates relevance and importance of the information to audience members.

Evaluation. Each time you present a PowerPoint presentation, reflect on the performance. What was the experience like? What worked? What could have been done better? What do the evaluations say about your PowerPoint, your presentation, and your performance? Listening to, accepting, and acting on the feedback of your audience helps you to refine and improve your presentation skills with each experience.

Discussion Boards

Discussion boards provide an electronic forum that allows participants to post a message that others can read and to which others can respond, enabling communication between members who can access the board at any time (Weisskirch & Milburn, 2003). There are a number of benefits e-learning has over traditional lectures, such as students being able to participate without having to travel to a particular place, the fact that students can reflect on forum messages that have been posted before responding to them, and that questions can be asked without students having to wait in turn to ask them.

On the Internet, discussion boards (also known as message boards, discussion forums, and online forums) were the original social media meeting places. As online bulletin boards where people with similar interests can discuss and debate various topics, discussion boards can enhance communication between you, your peers, and your instructors when used in conjunction with traditional on-campus courses, and can provide a forum for discussion in fully online courses.

During your course, you may be asked to use the discussion board to introduce yourself, to respond to instructor questions and reply to others, to formulate answers to case studies, or as part of a peer writing and review process. You may even be asked to lead a discussion.

Online discussions provide you with the opportunity to "think before you speak." You have time to reflect on what you want to say before you enter your response in the system. You are also able to view the responses and perspectives of all your classmates, which is not easily accomplished in a real classroom setting.

"NETIQUETTE" for Online Discussions

Respect fellow classmates. There is a great deal that we can learn from each other, but this cannot happen if students feel uncomfortable in class about speaking up (afraid that their ideas will be treated harshly or not "listened to" respectfully) or are worried about what will be said to them or about them once they do speak up. Make sure you do everything you can to make your classroom culture a comfortable learning environment for everyone in the class. You may have people from many different backgrounds in the class and people with many different levels of academic preparation. You should all feel comfortable and make each other comfortable with discussing the issues.

Use an appropriate tone of voice. Say what you need to say, but say it in an appropriate tone of voice—one that is respectful and calm. Sarcastic, heavily judgmental, or confrontational comments break down good will and create an inhospitable classroom atmosphere. Since this is a course that deals with ethics, among other issues, this is particularly critical. Bullying comments are inappropriate and unacceptable in this class. This is most important in the online component of the classroom, where tone of voice is often difficult to "read" from the language on screen (although the use of emotions helps reduce this difficulty in some ways).

Sample Discussion Board Participation Grade Guidelines

1. Consistently contributes to class discussion with summaries of required readings, questions, and comments. Frequently encourages others to contribute to the discussion by direct invitation and/or by expressions of interest in an acknowledgment of their comments. Attempts to parallel and summarize discussion points and/or resolves conflicting viewpoints. 4.0.

2. Contributes constructively in a number of sessions. Evidence of preparation for discussion of required readings. Offers a number of attempts to promote others' participation. 3.5.

3. Participates in some discussion. Contributes with focus on experiential background in lieu of required readings. 3.0.

4. Appears to be attending mindfully to class discussion. Participates actively only when directly asked for comment, rarely otherwise. 2.5.

5. Peripheral stance to class discussion. 2.0.

CHAPTER 9 REFLECTIVE QUESTIONS

1. Discuss your experience with technology in communication as a consumer, nurse, and student.

2. What has been your experience with simulation? How do you see simulation education as integrated into nursing education?

3. What are some things nurses can do to maintain caring in a highly technological care environment?

4. How might the role of the informatics nurse be implemented in your work setting?

5. Describe your experience with discussion boards (orientation, netiquette, ease of use, challenges).

CHAPTER 10

Professional Writing Skills in Nursing

OBJECTIVES

1. Identify characteristics of effective written communication.
2. Examine effective communication using SBAR (Situation, Background, Assessment, Recommendation).
3. Describe strategies in writing a research paper.
4. Explain the steps in conducting a literature search.
5. Discuss the PICOT method.

KEY TERMS

APA format

Citation

Communication

Incivility

Lateral violence

Literature search

Metacommunication

Nursing research

Patient population, intervention, comparison, outcome, time (PICOT)

STANDARDS

Safety		
Definition: Minimizes risk of harm to patients and providers through both system effectiveness and individual performance.		
Knowledge	**Skills**	**Attitudes**
Examine human factors and other basic safety design principles as well as commonly used unsafe practices (such as work-arounds and dangerous abbreviations). Describe the benefits and limitations of selected safety-enhancing technologies (such as barcodes, computer provider order entry, medication pumps, and automatic alerts/alarms). Discuss effective strategies to reduce reliance on memory	Demonstrate effective use of technology and standardized practices that support safety and quality. Demonstrate effective use of strategies to reduce risk of harm to self or others. Use appropriate strategies to reduce reliance on memory (such as forcing functions, checklists)	Value the contributions of standardization/ reliability to safety. Appreciate the cognitive and physical limits of human performance
Delineate general categories of errors and hazards in care. Describe factors that create a culture of safety (such as open communication strategies and organizational error reporting systems)	Communicate observations or concerns related to hazards and errors to patients, families, and the health care team. Use organizational error reporting systems for near miss and error reporting	Value own role in preventing errors
Describe processes used in understanding causes of error and allocation of responsibility and accountability (such as root cause analysis and failure mode effects analysis)	Participate appropriately in analyzing errors and designing system improvements. Engage in root cause analysis rather than blaming when errors or near misses occur	Value vigilance and monitoring (even of own performance of care activities) by patients, families, and other members of the health care team
Discuss potential and actual impact of national patient safety resources, initiatives, and regulations	Use national patient safety resources for own professional development and to focus attention on safety in care settings	Value relationship between national safety campaigns and implementation in local practices and practice settings

We cannot be truly human apart from communication . . . to impede communication is to reduce people to the status of things.

Paulo Freire
International educator, community activist

IMPORTANCE OF WRITTEN COMMUNICATION

Part of the nursing role is to educate others. This is often done through written handouts on health topics (for patients) and journal articles (for colleagues). It is essential that these educational materials be well written. No one is going to take us seriously if we have poor writing skills. In writing, we convey not only our meaning, but also our education and a sense of confidence that shows readers we have a firm grasp of the topic and that they can trust the information we provide.

I use my writing skills for all my documentation. I think that a well written-message gets a better response than a messy, dashed off scribble. It's important to value writing for documentation. While in computerized charting there [are] boxes to fill in, in many situations, they are not adequate to record the entire picture and you must use the narrative section.

Writing skills are very important, both in the medical record and in other communications. How much faith do you have in a nurse who cannot form a coherent sentence or spell the simplest words correctly?

Nursing student

This chapter reinforces the importance of written communication in nursing practice. Daily, nurses use writing skills to transmit information to a broad range of listeners. Effective writing promotes the use of critical thinking and analysis, and ensures that those individuals with whom the nurse interacts (clients, families, and colleagues) will understand what is being said.

E-mail communications with other members of the health care team necessitate proper writing skills. In the daily process of documenting in a client's chart, nurses use objective, professional, and succinct language to articulate the client's status and/or changes in condition. As evidence-based researchers, possessing technical writing skills and the ability to investigate and analyze areas of interest are important in sharing nursing information with colleagues. While research is further enhanced when outcomes are shared with colleagues, dissemination of written research generates new ideas in nursing. For those individuals in nurse leadership positions, writing skills are essential: staff meetings require clear and succinct agendas; evaluations, policies and procedures, and reports are frequently written for administrators, supervisors, or trustees; documentation here must reflect clear communication of circumstances and outcomes.

Professional writing in nursing is an important way to communicate with others, express ideas, present information, advance research, and teach others about the discipline of nursing. In writing, we open ourselves up to the possibility that our ideas are not consistent or compatible with our readers' values. We worry that our information negatively exposes us individually or professionally. In the end, however, we take these chances in the belief that the content of our words will ultimately help others (Lewis, 2009).

EFFECTIVE COMMUNICATION USING SBAR (SITUATION, BACKGROUND, ASSESSMENT, RECOMMENDATION)

Dr. Michael Leonard (Groff & Augello, 2003) describes the hazards of a "historical mindset"; that is, the belief that each person is educated as an expert and can handle any situation alone. This type of thinking actually hinders teamwork and team communication (Duncan & DePew, 2011). The environment of care has become so complex and intricate that one person is not always able to keep track of all the details of care. Leonard cites four limitations that affect caregivers: multitasking, short-term memory, fatigue, and stress. Together, these factors can contribute to performance and safety issues, as nurses "exceed the ability of our brains to manage and capture all the information" with the potential for devastating effects on clients. In order to work effectively as a team and provide safe, professional care, an effective communication method is needed. To address this challenge, Dr. Leonard developed the Situational Briefing model (2004), with the intent of improving communication among doctors, nurses, health care providers, and coworkers.

The nurse explains the present situation, describes the background, shares present assessment findings, and makes recommendations for solving the problem (Haig & Whittington, 2006). A significant contribution of SBAR is its distinctive acknowledgment of nurses' expertise. With this method, nurses are able to assert themselves, feel free to voice their concerns, and offer their recommendations to physicians and other members of the health care team.

Ineffective communication among health care team members can lead to adverse events for clients. The SBAR method has been proven instrumental in preventing negative patient outcomes (Dingley, Daugherty, Derieg, & Persing, 2008; Haig & Whittington, 2006; Leonard, Graham, & Bonacum, 2004). Because SBAR provides a standardized means for communicating in patient care situations, it is effective in bridging differences in communication styles. SBAR provides a common and predictable structure for communication and can be used in any clinical domain. SBAR also presents guidelines for organizing relevant information when preparing to contact another team member, as well as the framework for presenting the information, appropriate assessments, and recommendations (Dingley et al., 2008).

Either write something worth reading or do something worth writing.

Benjamin Franklin

THE NURSING RESEARCH PAPER

When writing papers, give yourself plenty of time to prepare for the work ahead. Read and reread the instructions for the paper. Ask yourself, "What is the purpose of this article?" Make it worth your efforts. Formulate any notes, ideas, or questions after reviewing the assignment, and consult your professor prior to beginning your work. Many nursing professors require that you submit your topic idea for approval prior to proceeding to the literature search.

Additionally, most nursing professors give detailed instructions on what is required in a writing assignment. Make sure you understand the expectations (scholarly resources, length of paper, content, criteria for grading). If a rubric is included in the assignment, follow it closely. You may want to develop an outline based on the specific rubric.

It is highly recommended that you discuss your ideas for your paper with your instructor. For example, are you to write a "report" on diabetes (probably not!), or is the focus on **nursing care** of the newly diagnosed diabetic with a focus on teaching to foster client compliance?

To avoid becoming overwhelmed, choose a finite subject. Refine your topic ("Teaching Foot Care Basics With the Newly Diagnosed Diabetic Client," rather than "Diabetes"). Ask yourself the following questions when starting the literature search: What current knowledge is out there regarding nursing practice on the topic I am studying? How many scholarly articles are required? Must they be nursing articles (national/international)? Can articles/resources from other disciplines be used? Are textbook references allowed? Most references must be no older than 5 years. Avoid resources such as Wikipedia and WebMD.

Choose a topic that is of interest to *you*, as well as one that is suited to the intent of the assignment. Often the topic you choose is the concept that you will carry with you as you advance in your nursing education. It could very well be the basis for your dissertation some time in the near/distant future.

Consult the university's library personnel. They provide a wealth of information for help with refining your search, accessing the appropriate references, and obtaining articles to include in the assignment. Refer to the American Psychological Association (APA, 2009) guidelines.

Find out if rough drafts are permitted; if so, take your professor up on this gift. It is a wonderful learning tool, helps a student understand what the "editor" is looking for, and ultimately makes a considerable difference in your final paper grade.

Finally, keep writing. The more you write, the better writer you will become.

Sample Research Paper With Instructor Feedback
(What grade would you give to this paper?)

Grading Rubric:	Possible Points
Introduction	10 points
Summary of the articles	30 points
Discussion of nursing care	30 points
Summary/Conclusion	10 points
Grammar, sentence structure	10 points
APA format	10 points

Labor Pain: Pharmacologic Versus Nonpharmacologic Interventions

One of the many challenges pregnant women face is the decision of how to manage their labor pain. Pain is highly subjective and patients tolerate and express pain in a variety of ways. Labor pain can be influenced by a number of factors, such as culture, anxiety, and environment. In addition, no two women have the same childbirth experience. As a result, patients need individualized birth plans that address their unique needs in order to effectively manage labor pain.

To devise a plan that works for her, the expectant mother needs to know all of her options. This includes education about pharmacologic and nonpharmacologic interventions. A lack of knowledge about the options for managing labor discomfort may increase anxiety and negatively affect what may be one of the happiest days of a woman's life. It is the nurse's role to ensure the patient is making an informed decision that is best for her. The nurse should make sure all of the patient's questions are answered, and provide any additional teaching when needed. This helps ensure the quality of the birthing experience.

The first article, by Weatherspoon (2011), provides a complete list of options for the management of labor discomfort. The goal is that childbirth educators will pass this information on to their patients. Emphasis is placed on using education to empower expectant mothers to make them feel in control during their pregnancy, labor, and delivery. A main point the author makes is that "the effects of acceptance, feelings of control, and attitude toward labor are probably related to the level of information the pregnant mother possesses" (Weatherspoon, 2011, p. 44). With that being said, childbirth educators should take the initiative to begin this education early on in the pregnancy, not when the patient comes in to deliver. The hypothesis is that this will help the patient feel more prepared, which in turn reduces anxiety and maximizes patient satisfaction.

The article also discusses how alternative methods are effective during labor. Relaxation techniques, such as deep breathing, may enhance natural endorphins that block pain receptors (Weatherspoon, 2011). Water therapy helps to manage pain by providing buoyancy to alleviate some of the pressure. Using forms of distraction such as guided imagery have been shown to reduce anxiety, lower blood pressure, and provide energy (Weatherspoon, 2011). Some women find comfort in a gentle stroking technique known as effleurage. Effleurage works by occupying sensory nerves, decreasing the intensity of pain (Weatherspoon, 2011). "Acupuncture or acupressure generates competing stimuli that block pain signals from reaching the brain" (Weatherspoon, 2011). These methods provide pain relief without the possible side effects that come with pharmacologic analgesia.

According to Weatherspoon (2011), "the epidural block remains the most common medical intervention for traditional labor analgesia" (p. 46). There is an increase in the satisfaction of using this method of analgesia since changes have occurred that give the patient more control. For example, patient-controlled epidural analgesia (PCEA) allows the mother to self-administer the medication via the epidural catheter, promoting patient autonomy (Weatherspoon, 2011). This article is significant to nursing care because when mothers are made aware of nonpharmacologic options, they can be explored during the initial stages of labor. If the patient decides they are ineffectively managing the pain, pharmacological methods can be tried. The point is that patients' autonomy is promoted by increasing their awareness.

The second article, by Taavoni, Abdolahian, Haghani, and Neysani (2011), is a study designed to evaluate the effectiveness of a birth ball on labor pain. It compares pharmacologic and nonpharmacologic pain management by stating that pharmacologic methods attempt to alleviate the physical sensation of labor pain, and nonpharmacologic methods attempt to prevent suffering by enhancing the psychological, emotional, and spiritual components of labor (Taavoni, Abdolahian, Haghani, & Neysani, 2011).

One nonpharmacologic intervention that was emphasized was the technique of positioning. Sitting upright or standing is thought to decrease labor pain, as opposed to the supine position. Because the use of a birth ball requires the patient to be in an upright position, it was hypothesized that birth balls can decrease labor pain (Taavoni et al., 2011).

The study used a sample of 60 primiparous volunteers from a large public hospital. They were between 18 and 35 years old, had cephalic presentation of the fetus, were between 38 and 40 weeks gestation, anticipated a normal birth, and had no history of infertility (Taavoni et al., 2011). The women were all in the active phase of labor and randomly assigned to either the birth ball group or the control group. The birth ball group was instructed to sit on the ball and rock their hips back and forth for a minimum of 30 minutes. The control group received routine care during labor, but no intervention for pain. Pain scores from 0 to 10 were recorded from each group after 30, 60, and 90 minutes. The results showed that the pain scores of women who used the birth ball were significantly lower than the pain scores of those in the control group (Taavoni et al., 2011). These results are significant to nursing care because patients in labor have many options to alleviate their pain. It is important that the nurse be cognizant of the variety of interventions so that they can be correctly utilized.

In conclusion, childbirth is a personal experience that is unique for all expecting mothers. The options for labor pain management are endless—effleurage, epidural, positioning, birth balls—and each of these methods approaches pain in a different way. It is important to teach pharmacologic and nonpharmacologic interventions to the patient during pregnancy in order to devise a successful birthing plan. This teaching will prevent knowledge deficits and enhance patient satisfaction. It is the nurse's role to participate in prenatal care in such a way that promises a successful delivery.

APA Quick Reference Guide

1. Margins: One inch on all sides (top, bottom, right, and left)

2. Font size: 12-point font type: Times New Roman, Courier, or similar font

3. Spacing: Double space the entire document, including: title page, abstract, body, references.

4. Alignment: Left justified, leaving the right margin uneven.

5. Paragraph: Indent one-half inch (1/2 inch).

6. Page numbering: Place the page number on the right margin, one-half to one inch from the top.

7. Page headers: A short version of the title should be on the same line, with five spaces to the left of the page number.

8. Hyphens: No hyphenation is allowed at the end of a line.

9. Italics: Use italics for book titles and periodical titles.

10. Capitalization: In the Reference list only, for book and article titles, capitalize only the first word, any proper nouns, and the first word of the subtitle.

11. Punctuation spacing: One space after all punctuation marks—commas, colons, semicolons, periods at the end of a sentence, periods after initials in personal names, and periods that separate parts of a reference citation.

Student Research Paper Checklist

1. Is the entire paper double spaced?

2. Are margins one inch?

3. Are the title page and references on separate pages and in the correct sequence?

4. Are all pages numbered consecutively beginning with the title page?

5. Is the title no more than 10 to 12 words?

6. Is the title page in the correct format?

7. Does each paragraph contain more than one sentence?

8. Are all references in the reference list also cited in the text?

9. Do text citations and references agree (spelling and date)?

10. Are journal titles spelled out?

11. Are the references arranged alphabetically by author surname or first important word of the title if no author is listed?

12. Are page numbers for all articles and book chapters included?

13. Is the spacing after punctuation correct?

14. Does the paper have an introduction, body, and summary?

15. Is the title repeated on the first page of the text (top of page 2)?

HOW TO CONDUCT A LITERATURE SEARCH

A literature search is an organized, well-planned examination of literature published on a topic of interest. A carefully structured literature search is the most effective and efficient way to locate comprehensive evidence on the subject being investigated. Evidence may be found in books, journals, government documents, and the internet (Harvard, 2007).

Creating a well-focused question is the first phase in a literature search. A focused question provides a better start with your search because it will help you determine appropriate keywords and limitations for your topic. When forming your question, make sure you are specific about your research topic. Things to consider are the type of client, the condition or situation you are researching, and the type of intervention or nursing procedure you are investigating.

THE PICOT METHOD

The PICOT method (Melnyk & Fineout-Overholt, 2010) is a mnemonic that encompasses the key components of a well-focused question. The question must identify: the patient problem; the treatment being considered for the patient; alternative treatment (if any); outcome to be achieved or avoided; and time period to be considered.

Patient population/patient condition of interest (P): How would the nurse describe a group of patients and what are the most important characteristics of the patients? This may incorporate the primary problem, disease, or coexisting conditions. Additionally, the sex, age, or race of a patient might be of relevance here.

Intervention of interest (I): Which main intervention is the nurse considering? What is to be done for the patient? What factors may influence the prognosis of the patient? Are there coexisting problems?

Comparison of interest (C): What is the main alternative to compare with the intervention? Is there a decision to be made between two medications or two diagnostic tests? The clinical question does not always need a specific comparison.

Outcome of interest (O): What can the nurse hope to accomplish, measure, improve, or affect? What are you trying to do for the patient? Relieve or eliminate the symptoms? Reduce the number of adverse events? Improve function or test scores?

Time (T): Is there a time element involved?

PICOT Example: "For the adult, acute care patient, what is the effect of hourly rounding compared to current practice on fall rates during hospitalization?"

THE LITERATURE SEARCH ITSELF

Information can come from many sources, in print or electronically. Books can be a good start on a topic, providing general or specific information. Make sure that any book you are planning to use contains current information and has been published within the last 5 years. Journal articles are excellent sources of information, as they are current and specific. Much of the cutting-edge research is published in journals, obtained using a citation database such as CINAHL.

A search strategy is a carefully devised plan to search for information. It is particularly important when using electronic citation databases, as it keeps the focus on the topic and within the boundaries of the search. Additionally, the search strategy takes the research question and breaks it into keywords or phrases.

To expand their search, some individuals use "truncate" and "wild card" techniques (Harvard, 2007). Truncation takes the base of a word to seek out words that begin with that base word: Nurs* = nurse, nurses, nursing, nursery. Wildcards are symbols used to replace one or more characters in a word: Wom?n = woman or women. To explore "and washing compliance by nurses," the following truncation and wild card methods and the following terms can be used: Handwash*; Complian*; Nurs*; Non-complian*; and Hand hygiene (p. 32).

"Boolean logic" connects terms in a literature search by using AND, OR, and NOT. *"AND"* narrows the search by ensuring terms appear in an article. For example, "handwash* AND complian* AND nurs*" would bring back articles that relate to hand washing and compliance and nursing, including all the truncated forms of the words.

"OR" expands the search by enabling any of the terms to appear in an article. It is also useful for linking synonyms. The example here of "hand wash* OR hand wash* OR hand hygiene" would bring back articles with hand washing and its synonyms.

"NOT" narrows the search by eliminating a term from your examination. If the term "handwash* NOT alcohol gel" is used, it would bring back articles on hand washing, but no articles on alcohol gels used in hand washing (Harvard, 2007, p. 33).

CHAPTER 10 REFLECTIVE QUESTIONS

1. When you sit down to write a paper, what do you do first?

2. What educational resources have you accessed in the past to help you write your paper?

3. Do you enlist the help of another individual to proofread your paper before submitting it to your professor? If so, has it been helpful? In what ways?

4. Have you taken advantage of your professor's offer to accept a rough draft prior to submission of your final paper? If so, has it been helpful? In what ways?

5. What has been your experience with written criteria, or "rubrics," which outline expectations for your paper?

References

Ackley, B., & Ladwig, G. (2011). *Nursing diagnosis handbook: An evidence-based guide to planning care* (9th ed.). St. Louis, MO: Mosby.

Agency for Healthcare Research and Quality. (n.d.). Retrieved from http://www.ahrq.gov

Aiken, L., Clarke, S., Sloane, D., Lake, E., & Cheney, T. (2008). Effects of hospital care environment on patient mortality and nurse outcomes. *Journal of Nursing Administration, 38*(5), 223–229.

Aiken, L., Havens, D., & Sloane, D. (2009). The Magnet Nursing Services Recognition Program: A comparison of two groups of Magnet hospitals. *Journal of Nursing Administration, 39*(7/8), 5–14.

Aiken, L. H., Clarke, S. P., Sloane, D. M., Sochalski, J. A., Busse, R., Clarke, H., . . . Shamian, J. (2001). Nurses' reports on hospital care in five countries. *Health Affairs (Millwood), 20*(3), 43–53.

American Association of Colleges of Nursing. (2004). *AACN position statement on the practice doctorate in nursing.* Washington, DC: Author.

American Association of Colleges of Nursing. (2006). *The essentials of doctoral education for advanced nursing practice.* Washington, DC: Author.

American Association of Colleges of Nursing. (2008a). *The essentials of baccalaureate education for professional nursing practice.* Washington, DC: Author.

American Association of Colleges of Nursing. (2008b). *Position statement on the preferred vision of the professoriate in baccalaureate and graduate nursing programs.* Washington, DC: Author.

American Association of Colleges of Nursing. (2012). *Nursing shortage fact sheet*. Retrieved from http://www.aacn.nche.edu/media-relations/NrsgShortageFS.pdf

American Nurses Association. (2001). *Code of ethics for nurses with interpretive statements*. Washington, DC: American Nurses Publishing.

American Nurses Association. (2004). *Nursing: Scope and standards of practice*. Washington, DC: Author.

American Nurses Association. (2005). *Code of ethics for nurses with interpretive statements*. Silver Spring, MD: Author.

American Nurses Association. (2006). *Assuring patient safety: Registered nurses' responsibility in all roles and settings to guard against working when fatigued* (Position Statement). Silver Spring, MD: Author.

American Nurses Association. (2008a). *About nursing: ANA's definition of nursing*. Washington, DC: Author. Retrieved from http://www.nursingworld.org

American Nurses Association. (2008b). *Nursing informatics: Scope and standards of practice*. Washington, DC: Author.

American Nurses Association. (2010). *Nursing: Scope and standards of practice* (2nd ed.). Silver Spring, MD: Author.

American Nurses Credentialing Center. (2013). *Magnet recognition program manual recognizing nursing excellence*. Silver Spring, MD: Author.

American Psychological Association. (2009). *Publication manual of the American Psychological Association* (6th ed.). Washington, DC: Author.

Anderson, L. W., Krathwohl, D. R., Airasian, P. W., Cruikshank, K. A., Mayer, R. E., Pintrich, P., . . . Wittrock, M. C. (2000). *A taxonomy for learning, teaching, and assessing: A revision of Bloom's taxonomy of educational objectives*. New York, NY: Pearson, Allyn & Bacon.

Armstrong, K., Laschinger, H., & Wong, C. (2009a). Workplace empowerment and magnet hospital characteristics as predictors of patient safety climate. *Journal of Nursing Administration, 39*(7/8 Suppl.), S17–24.

Armstrong, K., Laschinger, H., & Wong, C. (2009b). Workplace empowerment and magnet hospital characteristics as predictors of patient safety climate. *Journal of Nursing Care Quality, 24*(1), 55–62.

Austin, S. (2008). Seven legal tips for nursing practice. *Nursing, 38*(3), 34–39.

Ausubel, D. P. (2000). *The acquisition and retention of knowledge: A cognitive view*. Dordrecht, the Netherlands: Kluwer Academic.

Balzer-Riley, J. (2008). *Communication in nursing* (6th ed.). St. Louis, MO: Mosby.

Balzer-Riley, J. (2011). *Communication in nursing* (7th ed.). St. Louis, MO: Mosby.

Barkai, K., & Martin, P. (2006). Profile of settlement. *The Journal of the American Judges Association, 42*(3–4A), 34–39.

Bass, B., & Riggio, R. (2006). *Transformational leadership* (2nd ed.). Mahwah, NJ: Erlbaum.

Beauchamp, T. L., & Childress, J. F. (2009). *Principles of biomedical ethics* (6th ed.). New York, NY: Oxford University Press.

Benner, P. (1982). From novice to expert. *American Journal of Nursing, 82*(3), 402–407.

Benner, P. (1984). *From novice to expert: Excellence and power in clinical nursing practice*. Menlo Park, CA: Addison-Wesley.

Benner, P. (2004). Using the Dreyfus model of skill acquisition to describe and interpret skill acquisition and clinical judgment in nursing practice and education. *Bulletin of Science, Technology & Society, 24*(3), 188–219.

Benner, P., Sutphen, M., Leonard, V., & Day, L. (2010). *Educating nurses.* Stanford, CA: Jossey-Bass.

Benner, P., Tanner, C., & Chesla, C. (2009). *Expertise in nursing practice: Caring, clinical judgment, and ethics* (2nd ed.). New York, NY: Springer Publishing Company.

Billings, D., & Halstead, J. (2011). *Teaching in nursing: A guide for faculty* (4th ed.). St. Louis, MO: Elsevier.

Blais, K. K., & Hayes, J. S. (2011). *Professional nursing practice: Concepts and perspectives.* Boston: Pearson.

Blegen, M., Goode, C., Spetz, J., Vaughn, T., & Park, S. (2011). Nurse staffing effects on patient outcomes: Safety-net and non-safety-net hospitals. *Medical Care, 49*(4), 406–414.

Board of Higher Education and Massachusetts Organization of Nurse Executives. (2006, March 23–24). *Creativity and connections: Building the framework for the future of nursing education and practice.* A report from the Invitational Working Session, Worcester, MA. Retrieved from http://www.mass.edu/currentinit/documents/Nursing Creativity And Connections.pdf

Brooke, P. (2006). So you've been named in a lawsuit: What happens next? *Nursing, 36*(7), 44–48.

Buerhaus, P., Auerbach, D., & Staiger, D. (2009). The recent surge in nurse employment: Causes and implications. *Health Affairs, 28*(4), 657–668.

Burns, J. (1978). *Leadership.* New York, NY: Harper & Row.

Butts, J. B., & Rich, K. L. (2008). *Nursing ethics across the curriculum and into practice* (2nd ed.). Sudbury, MA: Jones & Bartlett.

Cant, R., & Cooper, S. (2010). Simulation-based learning in nurse education: A systematic review. *Journal of Advanced Nursing, 66*(1), 13–15.

Cara, C. (2003). Continuing education: A pragmatic view of Jean Watson's caring theory. *International Journal for Human Caring, 7*(3), 51–61.

Carr, J. (2006). *Healthy nurse: Escape burnout and discover the ultimate life/work balance.* Columbus, IN: Matilda.

Carroll, V. S. (2004). Nursing malpractice: Sidestepping legal minefields. *Quality Management in Healthcare, 13*(1), 93.

Chambers, D., Thompson, S., & Narayanasamy, A. (2013). Engendering cultural responsive care: A reflective model for nurse education. *Journal of Nursing Education and Practice, 3*(1), 70–81.

Chew, L. D., Bradley, K. A., & Boyko, E. J. (2004). Brief questions to identify patients with inadequate health literacy. *Family Medicine, 36*(8), 588–594.

Chinn, P. L., & Jacobs, M. K. (1987). *Theory and nursing: A systematic approach* (2nd ed.). St. Louis, MO: Mosby.

Chislett, V., & Chapman, A. (2005). *VAK Learning Styles Self-Assessment Questionnaire.* Retrieved from Tinyurl.com/vakquestionnaire

Christmas, K. (2009). 2009: The year of positive leadership. *Nursing Economics, 27*(2), 128–129, 133.

Clark, C., & Ahten, S. (2010). Beginning the conversation: The nurse educator's role in preventing incivility in the workplace. *RN Idaho, 33*, 9–10.

Clarke, S. P., & Aiken, L. H. (2003). Failure to rescue. *American Journal of Nursing, 103*(1), 42–47.

Connors, H., Weaver, C., & Warren, J. (2007). The perfect storm: Ratios, retirement and entry into practice. *Nursing Administration Quarterly, 31*(2), 129–133.

Croke, E. (2003). Nurses, negligence, and malpractice. *American Journal of Nursing, 103*(9), 54–63.

Cronenwett, L., & Sherwood, G. (2007). Current assessments of quality and safety education in nursing. *Nursing Outlook, 55*(3), 132–137.

Cronenwett, L., Sherwood, G., Barnsteiner, J., Disch, J., Johnson, J., Mitchell, P., . . . Warren, J. (2007). Quality and safety education for nurses. *Nursing Outlook, 55*(3), 122–131.

Cronenwett, L., Sherwood, G., Pohl, J., Barnsteiner, J., Moore, S., Sullivan, D., . . . Warren, J. (2009). Quality and safety education for advanced nursing practice. *Nursing Outlook, 57*(6), 338–348.

Daggett, L. M. (2008). A rubric for grading or editing student papers. *Nurse Educator, 33*(2), 55–56.

Dall'Alba, G. (2009). Learning professional ways of being: Ambiguities of becoming. *Educational Philosophy and Theory, 41*(1), 34–45.

Dayton, E., & Henriksen, K. (2007). Communication failure: Basic components, contributing factors, and the call for structure. *Joint Commission*

Journal on Quality and Patient Safety/Joint Commission Resources, 33(1), 34–47.

DeWan, S., & Ume-Nwagbo, P. (2006). Using the Neuman systems model for best practices. *Nursing Science Quarterly, 1*(19), 31–35.

Dey, S., & Kudumovic, M. (2010). The role of information technology in preventing medical errors. *Review of Global Medicine and Healthcare Research, 1*(1), 89–95.

Dingley, C., Daugherty, K., Derieg, M., & Persing, R. (2008). Improving patient safety through provider communication strategy enhancements. In K. Henriksen, J. B. Battles, M. A. Keyes, & M. L. Grady (Eds.), *Advances in patient safety: New directions and alternative approaches, Vol. 3: Performance and tools.* Rockville, MD: Agency for Healthcare Research and Quality.

Doheny, M., Cook, C., & Stopper, M. (1997). *The discipline of nursing: An introduction* (4th ed.). Stamford, CT: Appleton & Lange.

Drenkard, K. (2009). The Magnet imperative. *Journal of Nursing Administration, 39*(7/8), 1–2.

Dreyfus, H., & Dreyfus, S. (1980). *A five stage model of the mental activities involved in direct skill acquisition* (Operations Research Center report). Berkeley: University of California Press.

Duncan, G., & Depew, R. (2011). *Transitioning from LPN/VN to RN: Moving ahead in your career* (2nd ed.). New York, NY: Delmar.

Encinosa, W., & Bae, J. (2011–2012). Health information technology and its effects on hospital costs, outcomes, and patient safety. *Inquiry, 48*(4), 288–303.

Fadiman, A. (1997). *The spirit catches you and you fall down: A Hmong child, her American doctors, and the collision of two cultures.* New York, NY: Noonday Press.

Faila, K. R., & Stichler, J. F. (2008). Manager and staff perceptions of the manager's leadership style. *Journal of Nursing Administration, 38*(11), 480–487.

Falvo, D. (2011). *Effective patient education: A guide to increased compliance.* Sudbury, MA: Jones & Bartlett.

Fater, K. (2013). Gap analysis: A method to assess core competency development in the curriculum. *Nursing Education Perspectives, 34*(2), 101–105.

Fernandez, L., & Schillinger, D. (2009). *Literacy and patient care* (3rd ed.). Sudbury, MA: Jones & Bartlett.

Fineout-Overholt, E., Gallagher-Ford, L., Mazurek Melnyk, B., & Stillwell, S. B. (2011). Evidence-based practice, step by step: Evaluating and disseminating the impact of an evidence-based intervention: Show and tell. *American Journal of Nursing, 111*(7), 56–59.

Fineout-Overholt, E., Williamson, K. M., Gallagher-Ford, L., Melnyk, B. M., & Stillwell, S. B. (2011). Evidence-based practice, step by step: Following the evidence: Planning for sustainable change. *American Journal of Nursing, 111*(1), 54–60.

Forni, P. (2008). *The civility solution.* New York, NY: St. Martin's Press.

Frank, A. (1995) [1947]. Frank, O. H., Pressler, M. Eds. *Het Achterhuis [The Diary of a Young Girl—The Definitive Edition]* (in Dutch). Massotty, S. (translation). New York, NY: Doubleday.

Frankel, A. (2009). Nurses' learning styles: Promoting better integration of theory into practice. *Nursing Times, 105*(2), 24–27.

Frey, M., Sieloff, C., & Norris, D. (2002). King's conceptual system and theory of goal attainment: Past, present, and future. *Nursing Science Quarterly, 15*(2), 107–112.

George, J. (2011). *Nursing theories: The base for professional nursing practice* (6th ed.). Upper Saddle River, NJ: Prentice Hall/Pearson Education.

Gordon, M. (2010). *Manual of nursing diagnosis* (12th ed.). Sudbury, MA: Jones & Bartlett.

Groff, H., & Augello, T. (2003). From theory to practice: An interview with Dr. Michael Leonard. *Forum, 23,* 10–13.

Gustafson, D. L. (2005). Transcultural nursing theory from a critical cultural perspective. *Journal of Advances in Nursing Science, 28*(1), 2–16.

Hacker, D., & Sommers, N. (2012). *Rules for writers* (7th ed.). Bedford, MA: St. Martin's Press.

Haggard, E. (1963). Learning a process of change. In L. D. Crow & A. V. B. Crow (Eds.), *Readings in human learning* (pp. 7–19). New York, NY: McKay.

Haig, K., & Whittington, J. (2006). SBAR: A shared mental model for improving communication between clinicians. *Journal on Quality and Patient Safety, 32*(3), 167–175.

Halloran, E., & Thorson, M. (1996). Henderson's unique functions of nurses. In J. Fitzpatrick & A. Whall (Eds.), *Conceptual models of nursing: Analysis and application* (3rd ed.). Stamford, CT: Appleton & Lange.

Hart, M. (2010). A Delphi study to determine baseline informatics competencies for nurse managers. *Computers Informatics Nursing, 28*(6), 364–370.

Harvard, L. (2007). How to conduct an effective and valid literature search. *Nursing Times, 103*(45), 32–33.

Hendelman, W. (2009). *Medicine and professionalism.* Retrieved from http://www.med.uottawa.ca/students/md/professionalism/eng/about.html

Henderson, V. (1966). *The nature of nursing.* New York, NY: Macmillan.

Henderson, V. (1991). *The nature of nursing: Reflections after 25 years.* New York, NY: National League for Nursing.

Heuston, M., & Wolf, G. (2011). Transformational skills of successful nurse managers. *Journal of Nursing Administration, 41*(6), 248–251.

HIMSS Nursing Informatics Survey. (2007). Retrieved from http://www .himss.org

Hodge, M., Martin, C., Tavernier, D., Perea-Ryan, M., & Van Houten, L. (2008). Integrating simulation across the curriculum. *Nurse Educator, 33*(5), 210–214.

Hogan, M. (2007). *Prentice Hall reviews & rationales: Nursing fundamentals* (2nd ed.). Upper Saddle River, NJ: Prentice Hall/Pearson Education.

Horton, K., Maust, D., Mensik, J., & Scott, K. (2011). Development of a professional nursing framework: The journey toward nursing excellence. *Journal of Nursing Administration, 41*(6), 259–264.

Huber, D. (2006). *Leadership and nursing care management* (3rd ed.). Philadelphia, PA: W. B. Saunders.

Hunt, D. (2012, September/October). QSEN competencies: A bridge to practice. *Nursing Made Incredibly Easy, 10*(5), 1–3.

Institute of Medicine. (1999). *To err is human: Building a safer health system.* Washington, DC: National Academies Press.

Institute of Medicine. (2001). *Crossing the quality chasm: A new health system for the 21st century.* Washington, DC: National Academies Press.

Institute of Medicine. (2003). *Health professions education: A bridge to quality.* Washington, DC: National Academies Press.

Institute of Medicine. (2004). *Health literacy: A prescription to end confusion.* Washington, DC: National Academies Press.

Institute of Medicine. (2010). *The future of nursing: Leading change, advancing health.* Washington, DC: Committee on Quality of Health in America, Institute of Medicine.

Johnson, S., & Rea, R. (2009). Workplace bullying: Concerns for nurse leaders. *Journal of Nursing Administration, 39*, 84–90.

The Joint Commission. (2008). Behaviors that undermine a culture of safety. *Sentinel Event Alert, 40.* Retrieved from http://www.jointcommission. org/SentinelEvents/Sentineleventalert/sea_40.htm

The Joint Commission. (n.d.-a). *Health care at the crossroads: Strategies for addressing the evolving nursing crisis.* Retrieved from http://www .jointcommission.org

The Joint Commission. (n.d.-b). *Sentinel Event policies and procedures.* Retrieved from http://www.jointcommission.org/Sentinel_Event_ Policy_and_Procedures

Kaminski, J. (2010). Theory applied to informatics—Novice to expert. *Canadian Journal of Nursing Informatics, 5*(4), 967.

Katz, M. G., Jacobson, T. A., Veledar, E., & Kripalani, S. (2007). Patient literacy and question-asking behavior during the medical encounter: A mixed-methods analysis. *Journal of General Internal Medicine, 22*(6), 782–786.

Kawasaki, G. (2012). *Enchantment: The art of changing hearts, minds and actions.* New York, NY: Penguin Books.

Kearney-Nunnery, R. (2008). *Advancing your career: Concepts of professional nursing* (4th ed.). Philadelphia, PA: F. A. Davis.

Kerfoot, K. (2008). Bossing or serving?: How leaders execute effectively. *MedSurg Nursing, 17*(2), 133–134.

Kiger, A. (2004). *Teaching for health* (3rd ed.). Philadelphia, PA: Churchill Livingstone.

King, C., Hindenlang, B., Moseley, S., & Kuritz, P. (2008). Limited use of the human patient simulator by nurse faculty: An intervention program designed to increase use. *International Journal of Nursing Education Scholarship, 5*(1), 1–17.

Kleinman, A., Eisenberg, L., & Good, B. (1978). Culture, illness, and care: Clinical lessons from anthropologic and cross-cultural research. *Annals of Internal Medicine, 88*(2), 251–258.

Knowles, M. (1990). *The adult learner: A neglected species* (4th ed.). Houston, TX: Gulf.

Kolb, D. A. (1984). *Experiential learning: Experience as a source of learning and development.* New Jersey, NJ: Prentice Hall.

Krause, T. (2007). The effective safety leader: Leadership style and best practices. *The Magazine of Safety, Health and Loss Prevention, Occupational Hazards, 69*(12), 19.

Larkin, H. (2009). 10 years, 5 voices, 1 challenge. To err is human jump-started a movement to improve patient safety. How far have we come? Where do we go from here? *Hospital Health Network, 83*(10), 24–28.

Lavin, M., & Killeen, M. (2008). Tribute to Imogene King. *International Journal of Nursing Terminologies and Classifications: The Official Journal of NANDA International (United States), 19*(2), 44–47.

Leininger, M., & McFarland, M. (1991). *Culture care diversity and universality: A theory of nursing.* New York, NY: National League for Nursing Press.

Leininger, M., & McFarland, M. (2002). *Transcultural nursing: Concepts, theories, practices* (3rd ed.). Columbus, OH: Greyden Press.

Leininger, M. M. (1991). *The theory of culture care diversity and universality* (pp. 44–45). New York, NY: National League for Nursing.

Leininger, M. M., & McFarland, M. R. (2006). *Culture care diversity and universality: A worldwide nursing theory* (2nd ed.). Burlington, MA: Jones & Bartlett.

Leonard, M., Graham, S., & Bonacum, D. (2004). The human factor: The critical importance of effective teamwork and communication in providing safe care. *Quality and Safety in Health Care, 13,* 85–90.

Levine, K. (2012, May). When speaking the same language means speaking different languages. *Minority Nurse,* 45–47.

Lewin, K. (1951). *Field theory in social science.* New York, NY: Harper & Row.

Lewis, C. (2009). Are writing skills important for nursing and nurses? *Journal of Vascular Nursing, 27*(3), 69.

Lewis, M., & Lamb, G. (2011). A comprehensive model for teaching Quality and Safety Education for Nurses (QSEN) competencies. *Dean's Notes, 32*(5), 1–3.

London, F. (2008). Meeting the challenge: Patient education in a diverse America. *Journal for Nurses in Staff Development, 24*(6), 283–285.

Lower, J. (2012). Civility starts with you. *American Nurse Today, 7*(5), 21–22.

Luzinski, C. (2011). Transformational leadership. *Journal of Nursing Administration, 41*(12), 501–502.

MacQueen, J. (2007). Florence Nightingale's nursing practice. *Nursing History Review, 15,* 29–49.

Mahlin, M. (2010). Individual patient advocacy, collective responsibility and activism with professional nursing associations. *Nursing Ethics, 17*(2), 247–254.

Marquis, B., & Huston, C. (2009). *Leadership roles and management functions in nursing: Theory and application.* Philadelphia, PA: Lippincott Williams & Wilkins.

Maslach, C. (2003). *Burnout: The cost of caring.* Cambridge, MA: Malor Books.

Massachusetts Department of Higher Education. (2010). *Nurse of the future: Nursing core competencies. Creativity and connections: Building the framework for the future of nursing education and practice: The future is now.* Retrieved from http://www.mass.edu/currentinit/documents/NursingCoreCompetencies.pdf

Masters, K. (2014). *Role development in professional nursing practice.* Burlington, MA: Jones & Bartlett Learning.

McGuire, E., & Kennerly, S. (2006). Nurse managers as transformational and transactional leaders. *Nursing Economics, 24*(4), 179–185.

McHenry, D. M. (2007). A growing challenge: Patient education in a diverse America. *Journal for Nurses in Staff Development, 23*(2), 83–88.

McMahon, D. (2012). *Nursing standards of practice.* Houston, TX: McMahon & Associates.

McMasters, K. (2014). *Role development in professional nursing practice* (3rd ed.). Burlington, MA: Jones & Bartlett.

McNeill, B. (2012, January–March). You teach but does your patient really learn?: Basic principles to promote safer outcomes. *Tar Heel Nurse*, 9–16.

Melnyk, B. M., & Fineout-Overholt, E. (2010). *Evidence-based practice in nursing and healthcare: A guide to best practice* (2nd ed.). Philadelphia, PA: Lippincott Williams & Wilkins.

Melnyk, B. M., Fineout-Overholt, E., Gallagher-Ford, L., & Stillwell, S. B. (2011). Evidence-based practice, step by step: Sustaining evidence-based practice through organizational policies and an innovative model. *American Journal of Nursing, 111*(9), 57–60.

Melnyk, B. M., Fineout-Overholt, E., Stillwell, S. B., & Williamson, K. M. (2009). Evidence-based practice: Step by step. Igniting a spirit of inquiry: An essential foundation for evidence-based practice: How nurses can build the knowledge and skills they need to implement ERP. *American Journal of Nursing, 109*(11), 49–52.

Melo, D., & Carlton, K. H. (2008). A collaborative model to ensure graduating nurses are ready to use electronic health records. *CIN: Computers, Informatics, Nursing, 26*(1), 8–12.

Meyer, G., & Lavin, M. (2005). Vigilance: The essence of nursing. *The Online Journal of Issues in Nursing, 10*(1), 8.

Mills, S. (2007). *Adapt leadership styles to achieve objectives.* Retrieved August 13, 2013, from www.FireEngineering.com

Narayanasamy, A. (2002). The ACCESS model: A transcultural nursing practice framework. *British Journal of Nursing, 11*, 643–650.

National Council of State Boards of Nursing. (2004). *Regulation of advanced practice nursing.* Chicago, IL: Author.

National League for Nursing. (2008). *Preparing the next generation of nurses to practice in a technology-rich environment: An informatics agenda* (Position statement). Retrieved from http://www.nln.org/aboutnln/positionstatements/informatics_052808.pdf

National League for Nursing. (2010). *Outcomes and competencies for graduates of Practical/Vocational, Diploma, Associate Degree, Baccalaureate, Master's, Practice Doctorate and Research Doctorate programs in nursing.* New York, NY: Author.

National League for Nursing Accreditation Commission. (2011). *NLNAC accreditation manual,* Atlanta, GA: Author.

Neill, M., & Wotton, K. (2011). High-fidelity simulation debriefing in nursing education: A literature review. *International Nursing Association for Clinical Simulation and Learning, 7*(5), 161–168.

Neuman, B. (2001). On nursing theories and evidence. *Journal of Nursing Scholarship, 33*(2), 115–119.

Neuman, B., & Fawcett, J. (2011). *The Neuman systems model* (5th ed.). Upper Saddle River, NJ: Pearson.

New, N. (2010). Teaching so they hear: Using a co-created diabetes self-management education approach. *Journal of the American Academy of Nurse Practitioners, 22,* 316–325.

Nguyen, D. N., Zierler, B., & Nguyen, H. O. (2011). A survey of nursing faculty needs for training in use of new technologies for education and practice. *Journal of Nursing Education, 50*(4), 181–189.

Nightingale, F. (1969). *Notes on nursing: What it is and what it is not.* New York, NY: Dover. (Original work published 1860)

Nugent, P., & Vitale, B. (2011). *Fundamentals success: A Q&A review applying critical thinking to test taking.* Philadelphia, PA: F. A. Davis.

Office of Applied Studies, Substance Abuse and Mental Health Services Administration. (2008). *Results from the 2007 National Survey on Drug Use and Health: National findings.* Rockville, MD: U.S. Health and Human Services.

Office of the National Coordinator for Health Information Technology. (n.d.). Executive summary. Retrieved from http://www. os.dhhs.gov/health/executivesummary.html

Orem, D. (2001). *Nursing: Concepts of practice* (6th ed.). St. Louis, MO: Mosby.

Pearson, C., & Porath, C. (2009). *The cost of bad behavior.* New York, NY: Penguin Books.

Quality and safety education for nurses. (n.d.). Retrieved from http://www .qsen.org

Raiger, J. (2005). Applying a cultural lens to the concept of burnout. *Journal of Transcultural Nursing, 16*(1), 71–76.

Reising, D., & Allen, P. (2007). Protecting yourself from malpractice claims. *American Nurse Today, 2*(2), 1–3.

Rogers, C. (1969). *Freedom to learn.* Columbus, OH: Merrill.

Roy, C., & Andrews, H. (1999). *The Roy adaptation model* (2nd ed.). Stamford, CT: Appleton & Lange.

Saba, V., & McCormick, K. (2006). *Essentials of nursing informatics* (4th ed.). New York, NY: McGraw-Hill.

Saba, V., & Riley, J. (1997). Nursing informatics in nursing education. *Studies in Health Technology and Informatics, 61,* 185–190.

Schuster, P. (2008). *Concept mapping: A critical-thinking approach to care planning* (2nd ed.). Philadelphia, PA: F. A. Davis.

Selander, L. (2010). The power of environmental adaptation: Florence Nightingale's original theory for nursing practice. *Journal of Holistic Nursing, 28*(1), 81–88.

Selander, L., & Crane, P. (2012). The voice of Florence Nightingale on advocacy. *OJIN: The Online Journal of Issues in Nursing, 17*(1), Manuscript 1. doi:10.3912/OJIN.Vol17No01Man01.

Sherman, R., & Eggenberger, T. (2009). Taking charge: What every charge nurse needs to know. *Nurses First, 2*(4), 6–10.

Sherman, R., & Pross, E. (2010). Growing future nurse leaders to build and sustain healthy work environments at the unit level. *OJIN: The Online Journal of Issues in Nursing, 15*(1), Manuscript 1. doi:10.3912/OJIN.Vol15No01Man01

Sherwood, G., & Drenkard, K. (2007). Quality and safety curricula in nursing education: Matching practice realities. *Nursing Outlook, 55*(3), 151–155.

Shirey, M. R., & Fisher, M. L. (2008). Leadership agenda for change toward healthy work environments in acute and critical care. *Critical Care Nurse, 28*(5), 66–79.

Sitzman, K., & Eichelberger, L. (2010). *Understanding the work of nurse theorists: A creative beginning* (2nd ed.). Sudbury, MA: Jones & Bartlett.

Smedley, A. (2005). The importance of informatics competencies in nursing. *CIN: Computers, Informatics, Nursing, 23*(2), 106–110.

Stanley, K., Martin, M., Michel, Y., Welton, M., & Nemeth, S. (2007). Examining lateral violence in the nursing workplace. *Issues in Mental Health Nursing, 28*, 1247–1265.

Stichler, J. F. (2008). Succession planning: Why grooming their replacements is critical for nurse leaders. *Nursing for Women's Health, 12*(6), 525–528.

Stone, P., & Gershan, R. (2009). Nurse work environments and occupational safety in intensive care units. *Journal of Nursing Administration, 39*(7/8), 27–34.

Stubenrauch, J. (2007). Malpractice vs. negligence. *American Journal of Nursing, 107*(7), 63.

Sullivan, D. (2010). Connecting nursing education and practice: A focus on shared goals for quality and safety. *Creative Nursing, 16*(1), 37–43.

Sullivan, E., & Decker, P. (2005). *Effective leadership and management in nursing* (6th ed.). Upper Saddle River, NJ: Pearson Prentice Hall.

Taavoni, S., Abdolahian, S., Haghani, H., & Neysani, L. (2011). Effect of birth ball usage on pain in the active phase of labor: A randomized controlled trial. *Journal of Midwifery & Women's Health, 56*(2), 137–140.

Taylor, J., & Wros, P. (2007). Concept mapping: A nursing model for care planning. *Journal of Nursing Education, 46*(5), 211–216.

Technology Informatics Guiding Educational Reform. (2008). *The TIGER initiative: Evidence and informatics transforming nursing: 3-year action steps toward a 10-year vision.* Retrieved from http://www.tigersummit.com

Tomey, A. M., & Alligood, M. R. (1998). *Nursing theorists and their work*. St. Louis, MO: Mosby.

Trinkoff, A., Geiger-Brown, J., Brady, B., Lipscomb, J., & Muntaner, C. (2006). How long and how much are nurses now working? *American Journal of Nursing, 106*(4), 60–71.

Ulrich, B., Buerhaus, P., Donelan, K., Norman, L., & Dittus, R. (2009). Magnet status and registered nurse views of the work environment and nursing as a career. *Journal of Nursing Administration, 39*(7/8), 54–62.

United States Bureau of Labour Statistics, U.S. Department of Labor, *Occupational Outlook Handbook, 2012–13 Edition*. http://www.bls.gov./ooh/education-training-and-library/librarians.htm

Van Dyke, M. (2008). CNOs and CFOs team up to teach nurses business skills. *Nurse Leader, 6*(6), 17–25.

Vestal, V., Krautwurst, N., & Hack, R. (2008). A model for incorporating technology into student nurse clinical. *CIN: Computers, Informatics, Nursing, 26*(1), 2–4.

Vitello-Cicciu, J. (2010). Educating nurses: A call for transformation. *Journal of Nursing Administration, 40*(6), 261–262.

Walerius, T., Hill, P., & Anderson, M. (2009). Nurses' knowledge of Advance Directives, Patient Self-Determination Act, and Illinois Advance Directive Law. *Clinical Nurse Specialist, 23*(6), 316–320.

Warfield, J. (2008). Student usage of electronic medical record. *CIN: Computers, Informatics, Nursing, 26*(1), 12–13.

Warren, J., & Connors, H. (2007). Health information technology can and will transform nursing education. *Nursing Outlook, 55*(1), 58–60.

Watson, J. (1999). *Postmodern nursing and beyond*. Toronto, ON: Churchill Livingstone.

Watson, J. (2005). *Caring science as a sacred science*. Philadelphia, PA: F. A. Davis.

Watson, J. (2008). *The philosophy and science of caring*. Boulder: University Press of Colorado.

Weatherspoon, D. (2011). Current practices in easing discomfort from labor and delivery: Alternative and medical practices. *International Journal of Childbirth Education, 26*(4), 44–48.

Weberg, D. (2010). Transformational leadership and staff retention: An evidence review with implications for healthcare systems. *Nursing Administration Quaterly, 34*(3), 246–258.

Weisskirch, R. S., & Milburn, S. S. (2003). Virtual discussion: Understanding college students' electronic bulletin board use. *The Internet and Higher Education, 6*, 215–225.

Wolf, G., Triolo, P., & Ponte, P. (2008). Magnet recognition program: The next generation. *Journal of Nursing Administration, 38*(4), 200–204.

Xu, P. (2012). Using teach-back for patient education and self-management. *American Nurse Today, 7*(3), 2.

WEB REFERENCES AND RESOURCES

http://www.jointcommission.org/assets/1/18/health_care_at_the_cross-roads.pdf

http://www.jointcommission.org/assets/1/18/RWJ_Future_of_Nursing.pdf

http://www.jointcommission.org/assets/1/23/jconline_Aug_1_12.pdf

http://www.nchealthliteracy.org/toolkit/tool5.pdf

http://www.wisc.edu/writing/Handbook/DocAPA.html

http://www.lib.usm.edu/help/style_guides.html

http://owl.english.purdue.edu/handouts/research/r_apa.html

Index